Why Diet and Exercise Fail

How Current Research Contradicts Conventional Wisdom about Weight Loss

By Daniel Matthew Korn

Author's Note: This book is not meant to replace the care of a medical doctor. Any condition, particularly a condition that requires a diagnosis, requires the attention of a physician. The author has done his best to present up-to-date and accurate information in this book, but he cannot guarantee that the information in this book applies to your situation. This book is sold with the understanding that the publisher and the author are not rendering professional medical services. If expert medical assistance is needed, the services of a competent doctor should be sought.

Edited by Sharon Ruth Korn

Cover art by Alison Vallocchia

ISBN 978-0-615-29008-9

Visit the author's website at: www.whydietandexercisefail.com

Contents

Acknowledgements

This book was greatly improved by the editing of my mother, Sharon Ruth Korn, and she has my deep appreciation for her efforts. As I was growing up, her commitment to having me improve my writing frequently included the admonition, "Remember, some day you may want to write a book." It turns out she was right. I would also like to thank my friend, Chris Grow, who looked at my research notes and convinced me to try to get them published. He was the first person to believe in this effort.

Morris Rosenthal of Foner Books provided me with almost all of the information I needed to market and publish this book, along with recommending the web editor for designing the book's internet site. Chris Grow, Corey Missimore, Daniel Robins, Michael Whitaker, Nitzy Tamir, Netta Denes, Noa Issler, and Shelley Davidescu listened to ideas for different sections of the book, shared their experiences, and played devil's advocate against my arguments. Noa reviewed a partial draft and convinced me to complete the book when I thought I didn't have time. Netta's observations led to much of the research on the implications of genetic diversity.

Last, but not least, this book would not have been written if it were not for Mr. Jonathan Davis and the Interdisciplinary Center Herzliya (IDC), the Israeli university of which he is vice president. I would like to thank the IDC for being so accommodating and welcoming to foreign students who do not speak Hebrew. It is the experience of getting a degree in Israel, where I have seen its relatively low rate of childhood and teenage obesity despite high consumption of sugars and fats, that has led to the research for this book. The university program offering degrees taught in English has been one of the most interesting experiences of my life, both because I have met people from every part of the world and because I have become intimately familiar with a region that is a mystery to most Americans. I would like to thank Mr. Jonathan Davis for convincing me to have that experience and the Interdisciplinary Center Herzliya for making it possible.

Introduction

The United States of America was the source of most of the innovations of the 20th century. It was the first country to mass produce automobiles, to invent computers and the internet, to place a man on the moon, and to develop the world's dominant military technology. Currently, in the 21st century, we worry that we are losing our ability to produce and manufacture the innovations of the future, but a trip overseas quickly dispels that notion.

Visiting Jerusalem, I am about as far away from the city where I grew up, San Diego, California, as it is possible to get, literally on the other side of the world. Even so, in Jerusalem, at my favorite restaurant here, I can see Heinz Ketchup and Mustard. Business people work on Dell computers. Down the road is a General Motors dealership. The cash register here is made by IBM. Local cinemas have more movies from Hollywood than from Europe or Israel. People don't realize how much the U.S. makes and sells overseas until they take a trip abroad. The view in Madrid, Paris, or Jerusalem is quite similar in this regard.

This book is a product of my travels overseas. Two years ago, I was living in the Washington, D.C. area. I was working for a consulting company that was using computer technology to improve the drug development process and the quality of care in hospitals—technology that is literally life-changing. I realized that technological innovation had a tremendous untapped ability to benefit our health and our medical knowledge in ways that had not yet even begun to be explored. I wanted to participate in this innovation; it was the thing that made me feel at my best.

Perhaps it was living near Washington, D.C., a city that lives and breathes foreign affairs, or perhaps it was working with people from around the world, but when I was ready to learn more about the technology I was helping to develop, I decided to study abroad. With my first two degrees, I hadn't considered studying overseas, and I was impressed by the insights of my colleagues who had. Israel was one of the more interesting places whose universities accepted students who spoke only English. After a trip to San Diego to say goodbye to family and friends, I was off.

The distance between San Diego and Israel is large, figuratively and literally. There are no direct flights from San Diego to Israel. It takes two days and at least two flights to get there, and by the time you finally land you are exhausted. Then you have to go though customs, and then you drive to your final destination. In my case, that meant a car trip up through the winding and narrow road to the top of the mountain on which Jerusalem sits.

One of the first things you may notice as an American in Jerusalem is that there are an awful lot of teenage girls carrying machine guns with grenade launcher attachments. They seem to stand out more than the young men who are similarly armed. Then, after their weapons fade to become part of the scenery, you may notice how thin all of those well-armed young people are. This is in a country in which you cannot find a gym other than in a hotel, in which people drive everywhere, books are sold from vending machines, and people work at sedentary jobs in office buildings. The national snack is deep fried, ice cream is the favorite way to keep cool in the desert heat, and pastries are everywhere. The people of Israel do not seem particularly health conscious, yet childhood and teenage obesity is not a major issue.

The thinnest visiting American student wasn't so lean as the fattest Israeli. This was not due to genetics, because Americans who came to visit their Israeli cousins were built just like other Americans. How was it that these Israeli teenagers, who drank beer, ate pizza and pastries, and didn't work out stayed so much thinner than my fellow American students who tried to exercise and to avoid foods which were considered fattening? What was the secret of these Israeli students, who were so much thinner than their American and European counterparts?

I started asking the Israelis about their diet. This was not considered impolite, but it was seen as a rather strange line of questioning for an American visitor to pursue. "You don't want to know about the fence?" "No," I replied, "we have a border fence where I grew up as well." "You don't want to know about the terrorism?" "No," I replied again, "one of my friends was a passenger on the first plane that flew into the World Trade Center, so I am familiar with terrorism. What I want to know is why it is that you are all so thin." However, I soon realized that even the Israelis did not know why.

The Israelis assumed that we Americans must be eating junk food constantly, while at every meal we shared they offered me something deep fried or laden with sugar. It was amazing. How did they do it? It became my passion, and almost my obsession, to figure out their secret. Once I had found the answer, every spare moment I could find was consumed by writing this book.

In a sense, my original idea was correct. I knew that technology was going to massively improve our health and medical knowledge. At the time, I was thinking in terms of implementing electronic health records and unlocking the genome. Yet this book could not have been written without the development of advanced search algorithms to sort through large amounts of research papers and databases with information on food consumption all over the globe. The book could not have been distributed or marketed before the invention of the internet. In that sense, this book is a product of technology's ability to expand our medical knowledge and improve our health.

Part I: Rethinking Conventional Wisdom

"Tell me and I'll forget, show me and I may remember, involve me and I'll understand." -*Ancient Chinese Proverb*

It is unlikely that this is the first book about weight loss that you have ever read. Most of those books try to explain why their method works better than all the others. This book is going to take a very different approach to helping you lose weight. It is going to start by examining weight loss techniques that do not work. Since we want to know what does work, studying the diet techniques that do not work may seem to be a strange place to start. Consider this: Americans spend tens of billions of dollars every year on diet books, diet products, and gym memberships. In spite of this massive yearly investment aimed at achieving weight loss, every year more of us become overweight.

We are surrounded by people who are selling weight loss techniques that do not work. To enable us to be better judges of weight loss claims, it will be helpful to review research on the effectiveness of different popular diet techniques. This is going to help us avoid wasting time and effort on diets that are doomed to fail. We have to be detectives and find the unseen clues that are going to lead to success in cracking the mystery of how to lose weight and keep it off.

We would do well to follow the advice of the great fictional detective Sherlock Holmes, who said, "Once you eliminate the impossible, whatever remains, no matter how improbable, must be the truth." The first part of this book is about eliminating the impossible—the methods that are not going to lead to success in solving our mystery. Once we eliminate those diets and weight loss techniques that do not work, we can see what remains and try to use it to understand the truth of why weight gain occurs and how we can more effectively lose weight and keep it off. Now let's begin our search!

Exercise and Weight Loss

It is almost universally assumed that, if we get enough physical activity in our daily lives and eat properly, we are likely to be lean and healthy. We worry that children spend too much time watching television and playing computer games. However, even people who have jobs that are just as physically active as those typical of workers hundreds of years ago are becoming overweight in large numbers. We need to reexamine the link between exercise and weight maintenance or weight loss.

Body Mass Index

To track changes in obesity over time, we need a way of measuring to what degree people are overweight. The measurement most frequently used by scientists studying obesity is the Body Mass Index (BMI). It is a ratio calculated by dividing a person's weight in kilograms by the square of his or her height in meters. A score of 25 to 29.9 is generally considered to be overweight, 30 to 39.9 obese, and 40 or over severely obese. These scores are not perfect, and they can incorrectly classify athletic men with a large amount of muscle mass but very little fat as overweight. However, the BMI has been in use longer than other measurements such as body fat percentage or the waist-to-height ratio, and it is still the measurement most frequently used in obesity studies.

The History of Weight Gain

Consider this quote from "The Early History of the

President's Council on Physical Fitness":

> In December, 1953, Dr. Hans Kraus, M.D. . . . claimed that the affluent lifestyle of 20th century America was making life so easy and effortless that American adults and children were rapidly losing muscle tone . . . . [Americans] needed to engage in regular exercise to attain a state of physical fitness comparable to that of earlier times when Americans walked for transportation, worked on farms, and accomplished most activities through manual labor.[1]

President Eisenhower was justifiably concerned that the United States' economy and technology were leading to an American population that was less physically fit than its European counterparts. After all, Eisenhower was a veteran of World Wars I and II who was intimately aware of the importance of physical strength to an infantry soldier.

However, the number of adults in the U.S. who were severely obese (BMI ≥ 40) during his presidency in the 1950s was so small that it would not be tracked for another 30 years. The percentage of American adults who were obese (BMI ≥ 30) in the fifties was 9.7%,[2] over 70% less than the percentage today, which is 34% according to the National Center for Health Statistics. In

---

[1] Prager, Felice. "The Early History of the President's Council on Physical Fitness." Rewind the Fifties. 3/31/2009 <http://www.loti.com/sixties_history/The_Eisenhower_Years.htm>.
[2] "National Health and Nutrition Examination Survey." Centers for Disease Control and Prevention, National Center for Health Statistics. 4/11/2009 <http://www.cdc.gov/nchs/nhanes.htm>.

the 1900s, the number was about 1 in 150, or less than 1%.[1] Most of the obesity increase the United States experienced in the 20th century occurred long after work and travel were no longer a source of regular exercise for most people, not concurrently with the decrease in activity levels.

Physical Activity and Staying Thin

Actually, it is not certain that people in the United States are much less physically active than people in less technologically developed societies. In fact, a recent study shows that levels of energy expenditure of women in rural Nigeria and metropolitan Chicago are not that different. Yet, despite performing similar amounts of physical activity, the women in Nigeria are much thinner than the women in Chicago. More interestingly, even within each group of women, the ones who are the most active are not significantly thinner. Since they are not getting more exercise than their American counterparts, it must be that something other than exercise is keeping Nigerian women thin and giving the United States a high rate of people who are overweight.[2]

---

[1] National Institutes of Health, National Heart, Lung, and Blood Institute, "Clinical Guidelines on the Identification, Evaluation and Treatment of Overweight and Obesity in Adults," 1998.

[2] Ebersole, Kara E.. "Energy Expenditure and Adiposity in Nigerian and African-American Women." Obesity: A Research Journal. 3/31/2009 <http://www.nature.com/oby/journal/v16/n9/abs/oby2008330a.html#aff1>.

Physical Activity and Staying Fat

Since the Nigerian women are not more active than the women in Chicago, perhaps the lack of food is what keeps them thin. This leaves the possibility that exercise can help us stay lean when we are exposed to the modern Western diet. In our society, there are still jobs which involve a very high level of physical activity. While many crops are planted and harvested mechanically, most fruits and vegetables are still planted and picked by hand, as they have been for thousands of years. For this reason, the fruit and vegetable farms of my native state of California require massive amounts of labor.

These farming jobs are some of the hardest and lowest paying available in California. Teenagers and low income Americans would much rather work in retail or fast food jobs. Working on the farms involves staying outdoors all day and engaging in manual labor. There are very few tools, other than those that are manually powered. This is the intense nature of work that humans engaged in for thousands of years, during which our ancestors were all lean. If an increasingly sedentary lifestyle were responsible for the weight gain of the American population, we would expect agricultural workers to be the thinnest people in California. However, this is not the case. In fact, a study found that 81% of male agricultural workers and 76% of female agricultural workers were either overweight or obese.[1]

---

[1] Rodriguez, Michael. "Health of Migrant Farmworkers in California." California Research Bureau. 3/31/2009 <www.library.ca.gov/crb/03/05/03-005.pdf>.

We can conclude that physical activity level does not seem to keep Nigerian women thin, nor does it prevent California's agricultural workers from becoming overweight. Later, we are going to see that genetics play a role in allowing people to become overweight when they are exposed to the right conditions, but they are not the cause of obesity. Two people who get exactly the same diet and level of exercise will not necessarily weigh the same amount because of genetic differences, so one could argue that the women in Nigeria may have some genetic trait that allows them to stay thin despite a low physical activity level. However, this argument would predict that Nigerian women would stay thin when they immigrated to the United States, and this is not the case. Thus, physical activity and genetics are not the reason women in Nigeria are lean. There is something present in the United States that is not present in Nigeria, or is present only in small amounts, which is causing these women to become overweight when they immigrate.

Similarly, the ancestors of agricultural workers in California were all lean. Their physical activity level was not too different from what is experienced on farms today. Yet the ancestors were thin, while the descendants are becoming overweight. The only differences that can explain the rising level of obesity are the diets people eat and the environment in which they live.

While exercise may not be what is keeping people in Nigeria lean, and it is not preventing California's agricultural workers from becoming overweight, it is possible it can help people who are overweight become lean again in combination with diet. After all, we frequently hear that a combination of diet and exercise is the key to weight loss. So let us examine whether diet and exercise together are more effective than diet alone, jointly comprising the best method of weight loss.

Hoping to Lose Weight by Exercising

The United States is filled with gyms. For the most part, people are not going to those gyms because they want to be healthy; they are going because they want to be thin and toned. The prevailing wisdom says that eating fewer calories and burning even more through exercise will make us thin or keep us thin.

We saw that when the President's Council on Physical Fitness was established, Americans were already leading very sedentary lives. Yet, our lack of exercise had not caused us to become overweight the way we are now. So the idea that lack of exercise is responsible for weight gain does not take into account that Americans used to be much thinner without exercising strenuously or leading very active lives. A U.S. Government study of the largest and best controlled experiments studying the effects of exercise and diet concluded that:

> While physical inactivity appears [to correlate with] obesity, studies on the effectiveness of [exercise] in promoting weight loss have been less than encouraging. Because physical activity increases energy expenditure, it is reasonable to assume that the combination of diet plus exercise would be more effective than dieting alone for weight loss. A recent review of 13 controlled studies found that this is rarely the case. Only two of the 13 studies reported statistically significant differences in weight loss

from the diet plus exercise regimen compared to diet alone. The conclusion from this review was that '*...exercise does not significantly increase initial weight loss over and above that obtained with diet only.*'[1]

The study did find that exercise has positive health benefits. However, weight loss does not appear to be one of them. Lack of exercise does not seem to be the cause of weight gain, and exercising does not seem to lead to long-term weight loss. The belief that exercise is related to weight has caused many of us to engage in excess physical activity that we do not enjoy, which does not get us to our desired goal, and which can also lead to injury.

---

[1] Welk , Gregory J. and Steven N. Blair. "Physical Activity Protects against the Health Risks of Obesity." President's Council on Physical Fitness and Sports Research Digest. 3/31/2009 <http://www.fitness.gov/digest_dec2000.htm>.

Fat and Weight Loss

There are probably few things as likely to confuse a potential dieter as fat. After all, there is a highly vocal group of people who believe that the best diet is one that is high in protein and fat, while there is another group that claims fat should be avoided to lose weight, and there is a third group advocating for us to avoid "bad" fats and eat "good" fats.

So fat either causes, reverses, or may cause weight gain. These are, of course, mutually exclusive ideas. At most, one of them can be correct. While we cannot easily perform an experiment ourselves to test which is correct, we can look at real world data and other people's experiments. Even someone who does not have scientific knowledge or medical education can learn a lot just by looking at real world data.

The French Paradox

The idea that fat causes heart disease and weight gain is a relatively old one. That it was commonly believed is evidenced by the surprise the Irish physician Samuel Black expressed in 1819 on discovering the low rate of heart disease the French experience, despite diets high in saturated fats. This contradiction between the expected and actual results of the French diet on the citizenry of France became known as the "French Paradox."

Today the French still eat a diet high in all fats, including saturated fat. They are high consumers of red meat, cheese, butter, and cream, and they drink an average of 11.4 liters of alcohol per year, compared to 8.6 liters per year for Americans.

Despite its high fat diet and high rate of alcohol consumption, France still has a relatively low rate of heart disease.[1]

Some scientists have questioned that a paradox really exists, arguing that heart disease rates in France are high, but they are not being properly counted or reported. What is not in dispute is that, despite eating significantly more fat than Americans, the percentage of people who are obese (BMI $\geq$ 30) in France is less than a third of the percentage in the U.S.[2] Higher fat consumption is not keeping the French from being thinner than Americans, even while they exercise less and drink more alcohol. This is fairly strong evidence that eating fat does not necessarily make people fat. Of course, there is always the possibility that the French are thin because they have a gene that protects them from gaining weight. So let us look at a people who have stayed thin while eating a very high fat diet but who have gained weight upon adopting a lower fat diet.

The Inuit People

We can see echoes of Dr. Black's surprise in 1819 in the October 2004 issue of *Discover Magazine*. Perhaps invoking the French Paradox, the article about the Inuit asks, "How can people who gorge on fat and rarely see a vegetable be healthier than we

---

[1] "Core Health Indicators." World Health Organization Statistical Information System. 3/31/2009 <http://www.who.int/whosis/>.
[2] Spencer, Mimi. "Let them eat cake." The Observer. 4/04/2009 <http://www.guardian.co.uk/lifeandstyle/2004/nov/07/foodanddrink.features11>.

are?"[1] In almost two hundred years, the common assumption that fat causes obesity has not changed.

The Inuit, often called Eskimos in the United States, traditionally ate a diet that included walrus, ringed seal, bearded seal, beluga whale, polar bear, berries, and fireweed. The Inuit believed their diet kept them warm and strong. However, the main reason they consumed this diet was due to the fact that they had little choice. It is very difficult to grow food in the Arctic, although the Inuit do gather plants that are naturally available. Very few calories in the Inuit diet come from these plants. Overall, 75% of the diet's calories are from fat.

If a high fat diet caused obesity, we would assume that Inuit who gave up their traditional diet and shifted towards a comparatively lower fat Western diet would be thinner and healthier. However, exactly the opposite has been occurring. Those Inuit who have given up their traditional diet in favor of the Western diet have experienced obesity, diabetes, high blood pressure, and cardiovascular disease.[2]

This is even more convincing evidence that fat and meat consumption does not cause obesity. With the French, the argument can be made that there is a genetic cause for the low rate of obesity. Our genes certainly do not make us fat, but they

---

[1] Gadsby, Patricia. "The Inuit Paradox." Discover Magazine. 4/04/2009 <http://discovermagazine.com/2004/oct/inuit-paradox>.

[2] Dewailly, Eric. "n-3 Fatty acids and cardiovascular disease risk factors among the Inuit of Nunavik." American Journal of Clinical Nutrition. 4/04/2009 <http://www.ajcn.org/cgi/content/abstract/74/4/464>.

do allow us to become fat. One could argue that the French have a high prevalence of a gene that keeps them from putting on weight, but we know that this is not the case with the Inuit. The Inuit who maintain their traditional high fat diet remain lean. The Inuit who are gaining weight do so as their consumption of fat and meat decreases. Fat and meat cannot be the cause of their weight gain. Since both groups are living in the same area, environmental factors can be ruled out as well.

The High Fat Diet

In 1972, Dr. Robert Atkins, an American internist and cardiologist, released a book titled *Dr. Atkins' Diet Revolution*. Over the next 30 years, he wrote 14 more books, in which he claimed that it was not fat that was responsible for unhealthy weight gain, but refined carbohydrates.

Atkins believed that sugar, flour, and high-fructose corn syrup were responsible for the rise of metabolic disorders of the 20th century. He also felt that wrongly focusing on fat as the cause of weight gain had made the problem much worse.[1] His ideas were very controversial, but they were convincing to many people. At the height of his diet's popularity in 2004, over 10% of adults in North America were following it.[2] While conventional science was originally dismissive of Atkins, by attracting so many adherents he made the diet so mainstream that science could not

---

[1] Atkins, Robert C. *Dr. Atkins' Diet Revolution* Bantam, 1972

[2] Kaufman, Wendy. "Atkins Bankruptcy a Boon for Pasta Makers." National Public Radio. 4/04/2009 <http://www.npr.org/templates/story/story.php?storyId=4783324>.

ignore him. Several experimental studies were performed comparing his diet to more traditional diet programs. The results were mixed.

One study concluded that there was an advantage in weight loss over other diets, but it was due to a loss in water weight.[1] Another found no major benefit compared to traditional diets, with some harmful side effects.[2] However, what is most interesting is what was not reported as a result in the studies. People who were put on this very high fat diet did not gain weight. Many of them lost weight. Notably, these were people who were already overweight, which means they could not have been genetically prone to thinness.

These short-term studies show that dietary fat content, at least by itself, is not what is responsible for weight gain. This is a remarkable conclusion. However, the Atkins diet does not appear to hold the secret to weight loss, either. Between 2004 and 2005, the Atkins diet's popularity fell from over 10% of North American adults participating to closer to 2% because, despite achieving some results, most dieters did not reach their ideal weight. [3]

---

[1] "Carbs may be worse for heart than fatty foods." MSNBC. 4/04/2009 <http://www.msnbc.msn.com/id/15625548/>.

[2] Johnston, Carol S. "Ketogenic low-carbohydrate diets have no metabolic advantage over nonketogenic low-carbohydrate diets." American Journal of Clinical Nutrition. 4/04/2009 <http://www.ajcn.org/cgi/content/abstract/83/5/1055>.

[3] "Atkins diet." Wikipedia. 4/04/2009 <http://en.wikipedia.org/wiki/Atkins_diet>.

Fat Quantity Is Not the Problem or the Solution

In the 1950s, people living in Europe, and especially in Crete, had almost no obesity. This was despite the fact that over 40% of their caloric intake was from fats. The main fat in their diet was olive oil.[1] This gave rise to another popular diet, the Mediterranean diet, which has been less controversial than the Atkins diet.

Olive oil is promoted as a "good" fat, while saturated fats from animals are "bad" fats. Although this has been uncontroversial, it has unfortunately not been a complete theory of weight control. Today the people of Crete eat amounts of olive oil comparable to levels of consumption in the 1950s, but now over half of them are overweight. This is despite the fact that there has been no change in olive oil consumption.

When we put all of these examples together, they make a fairly strong case that the overall level of fat consumption cannot explain the modern increase in the prevalence of obesity. The French are eating high levels of fat but remaining relatively thin. The traditional Inuit diet was 75% fat, but the Inuit remained thin, developing high rates of heart disease, obesity, and diabetes only when they adopted the relatively lower fat Western diet. Overweight followers of the Atkins diet restricted themselves to an almost purely protein and fat diet and were even shown to lose

---

[1] Kafatos, A., A. Diacatou, G. Voukiklaris, et al. 1997. "Heart disease risk-factor status and dietary changes in the Cretan population over the past 30 years: the Seven Countries Study." American Journal of Clinical Nutrition 65 (6):1882-86.

some weight. A diet rich in olive oil has not prevented the people of Crete from becoming overweight.

Collectively, these examples make clear that the level of fat consumption by itself cannot explain why people become overweight, although they do not rule out the idea that some fats are helpful and some are harmful. Yet, from the Irish physician Samuel Black expressing surprise at the low level of heart disease in the French, to the modern medical establishment's horror over the Atkins diet, to the surprise at the low levels of cardiovascular disease, diabetes, and obesity of the Inuit on their high fat diet, the belief that all fat consumption leads to weight gain is still accepted unconditionally by many. If this is really not the case, how is it possible that we could be so wrong for so long? Doesn't there have to be something to explain away these paradoxes?

Correlation Is Not Cause

What has really happened here is that we have fallen into a common error in understanding statistical data. We have wrongly assumed that, just because two things are associated, one causes the other. If we look at the fat consumption of most countries and the rate of people who are overweight in those countries, as fat consumption goes up, people tend to be more overweight. It has seemed obvious to most people who have observed this correlation that fat consumption was what was causing people to be overweight.

However, the vast majority of fat consumption comes from meat and dairy products. In comparing the amount of fat in the diets of different countries, the correlation between animal product consumption and fat consumption is over 90%.[1] As countries become richer, on average their people consume more meat and dairy products, most of which are derived from modern farming techniques. The type of fat contained in most of today's meat and dairy products is very different from what it was traditionally. So it isn't just that as countries eat more fat their populations become fatter. As countries become richer, many of their people eat more meat and dairy products that are more available, as well as different in fat content, because of modern farming techniques. We have been confusing the effects of high fat consumption with the effects of the increased wealth and the changes in agricultural techniques that have helped to make high fat consumption possible.

In the 19th century, meat consumption was very low compared to today. Meat was considered a prestige food in Europe, Asia, and Latin America, with the rich eating much more meat than the poor.[2] In 21st century America and Europe, almost all of us are rich by comparison, despite current economic woes. Increased wealth has gone hand in hand with weight gain in some countries, including the United States, the United Kingdom, Mexico, and Greece.

People in other countries, such as France, Norway, Japan, and South Korea have stayed quite thin. The rate of severely overweight people in Japan and Korea is over 90% less than in the United States. In France, it is over 70% less than in the United

---

[1] Campbell, T. Colin. *The China Study*. BenBella Books, Inc., 2005. p. 83.

[2] Friedman, Jonathan. *Consumption and Identity: Workshop on commodities and cultural strategies*. Taylor & Francis, 1994. p. 119.

States. The people in these countries have maintained leaner bodies despite living in developed, urban and highly technologically advanced societies.

A large amount of weight loss research has been based on examining the differences in the quantity of fat consumed between countries. However, the idea that even certain types of fat are responsible for weight gain is incomplete. If the amount or type of fat consumed were the sole cause of weight gain, all of the low fat diets of the 20th century would be effective, and people on the Atkins diet would all have gained weight.

Carbohydrates and Weight Loss

If fats do not cause weight gain, another culprit must be the cause. The theory that carbohydrates cause weight gain was popularized by Dr. Robert Atkins. His high fat, high protein diet has fallen out of favor, but there are still many diets advocating reducing or eliminating certain kinds of carbohydrates. While eliminating all carbohydrates is no longer in vogue, refined carbohydrates, particularly sugars, are still viewed as unhealthy.

Carbohydrates fill numerous roles in living organisms. They are involved in the storage and transportation of energy, they are used to build cartilage in animals, and they play a role in the immune system, fertilization, and blood clotting. The reason people can live on high fat diets like that devised by Dr. Atkins is because humans have the ability to make the carbohydrate glucose out of protein and fat.[1] The brain and nervous system require this glucose for energy.

Refined Carbohydrates

Clearly, we cannot say that all carbohydrates are bad or even that all sugars are bad. The body requires sugars to survive, even manufacturing them when they are not consumed. That having been said, the carbohydrates we eat today are different from those we ate historically.

---

[1] "Is dietary carbohydrate essential for human nutrition?" - Westman 75 (5): 951 - American Journal of Clinical Nutrition

Today we are processing grains with machinery that removes the bran and germ from the whole grain. This processing, or refining, of carbohydrates has increased the speed with which food is able to raise blood sugar. Refined carbohydrates are non-whole grain foods like white bread, white rice, and pasta and baked goods made with white flour.

There are scientists who believe that, by eating more foods that quickly raise our blood sugar, we are harming our bodies' ability to manage our blood sugar. Their theory is that weight gain is caused by the body's reaction to these sharp changes in blood sugar, and that the key to weight loss is to avoid foods that cause rapid changes in blood sugar. While this idea is still controversial among scientists,[1] new ideas usually are controversial. Let us examine the evidence.

Thailand

Thai meals always include rice. The Thai term for something served with rice literally means "not rice." In the 1950s, a group of researchers from Cornell University did a study of the diet of a small rice-growing village. They found that both the rich and the poor got about 80% of their calories from rice. Almost all of this rice was processed white rice, a refined carbohydrate, with a few percent being only partially refined rice that was being milled in the villagers' homes. The remaining

---

[1] Roth, Ronald. "Simple, refined, complex sugar/carbs, Glycemic Index & negative health effect." Cellular Nutrition. 4/04/2009 <http://www.acu-cell.com/gi.html>.

calories came from unrefined carbohydrates and animal sources.[1] The main health problems the villagers experienced were a deficiency of vitamin B, which is present in unprocessed rice but is removed by processing, and parasitic infections due to poor sanitary conditions. Obesity was not mentioned as a health concern.

At the national level in Thailand, consumption of white rice, a refined carbohydrate, still makes up between 70% and 80% of the calories in the diet.[2] In the United States, calories from carbohydrates make up about 50% of the diet.[3] The percentage of Thai adults who are obese (BMI $\geq$ 30) is less than 6%.[4] This is more than 80% less than the rate in the United States and a far lower rate than that of any European country. More interestingly since genetics can't explain the difference, in Thailand the rate of obesity is highest in the urban areas. There nutrition is more similar to the Western diet; consumption of refined carbohydrates is lower than in the rural areas. Since obesity in Thailand is highest where consumption of refined carbohydrates is lowest, refined carbohydrates cannot be the cause of obesity in that country.

---

[1] Hauck, Hazel M. et al, *Food Habits and Nutrient Intakes in a Siamese Rice Village, Studies in Bang Chan*, Cornell University, Ithaca, New York, 1958

[2] Gershoff, Stanley N. "Amino acid fortification of rice studies in Thailand." American Journal of Clinical Nutrition. 4/04/2009 <http://www.ajcn.org/cgi/reprint/28/2/170.pdf>.

[3] "National Health and Nutrition Examination Survey." National Center for Health Statistics. 4/04/2009 <http://www.cdc.gov/nchs/nhanes.htm>.

[4] Pongchaiyakul, C. "Defining obesity by body mass index in the Thai population: an epidemiologic study." PubMed. 4/04/2009 <http://www.ncbi.nlm.nih.gov/pubmed/16837420>.

Juice

While fruit juice is filled with many nutrients, calorically it is almost pure sugar. For this reason, people who believe that sugar is responsible for weight gain discourage the drinking of fruit juice. In 2006, the Minnesota Medical Association asked the federal government to remove fruit juices from its subsidized meal program that serves about 8 million low-income Americans.[1]

However, we should remember that juice was available long before the modern period. The Greeks fermented grapes to make wine, and certain Zoroastrian Persians ate a diet that consisted almost completely of fruit and fruit juice.[2] Despite the fact that fruits and fruit juices have been consumed for thousands of years, until the 20th century there were no examples of societies in which even one percent of the population was overweight. Not surprisingly, in the same year the Minnesota Medical Association made its request to the federal government, a study was published showing no correlation between consumption of pure fruit juice and weight gain.[3] Other studies have reached similar conclusions.[4]

---

[1] Lerner, Maura. "Fruit juice is a target in the war on obesity." Star Tribune. 4/04/2009 <http://www.startribune.com/lifestyle/health/11345236.html>.

[2] "History of Iran." Iran Chamber Society. 4/04/2009 <http://www.iranchamber.com/history/articles/sassanids_religious_turmoil.php>.

[3] Nicklas, Theresa A. "Association Between 100% Juice Consumption and Nutrient Intake and Weight of Children Aged 2 to 11 Years." Archives of Pediatrics & Adolescent Medicine. 4/04/2009 <http://archpedi.ama-assn.org/cgi/content/abstract/162/6/557>.

[4] "Drinking juice not associated with overweight and obesity in children." News-Medical.Net. 4/04/2009 <http://www.news-medical.net/?id=38842>.

Wrongly Accused

So why are carbohydrates suspected of causing weight gain, if the population of a country that eats more carbohydrates can be thinner than one which eats fewer, and low carbohydrate diets haven't resulted in long-term weight loss? Why are sugars suspected of leading to weight gain, if drinking sugar in the form of juice has not been linked to weight gain? It is because over the last forty years Americans have been getting more of their calories from simple sugar, a carbohydrate. During this time, the rate of Americans who are severely overweight has tripled.

While the two factors are correlated, it does not appear that one causes the other. In addition to the previous examples, a three-year study published in 2002 by the National Academy of Sciences concluded, "There is no clear and consistent association between increased intake of added sugars and [body weight]."[1] Neither refined carbohydrates nor simple carbohydrates cause weight gain.

Despite real world examples and scientific studies, a large percentage of the public remains convinced that refined carbohydrates and sugars cause weight gain. So great is the suspicion of sugar that it is almost impossible to find a major restaurant in the United States that does not serve diet soda. People would rather have this nutritionally empty drink, filled with chemicals and stimulants, created with an artificial sweetener, than fruit juice that contains sugar. It is thus highly

[1] Dietary Reference Intakes. Washington, D.C.: National Academies Press, 2004. p. 96

ironic that, while juice isn't correlated with weight gain, diet soda consumption is.[1]

[1] DeNoon, Daniel J. "Drink More Diet Soda, Gain More Weight?" WebMD. 4/04/2009 <http://www.webmd.com/diet/news/20050613/drink-more-diet-soda-gain-more-weight>.

Genetics and Weight Loss

When we look at people who are overweight today, they tend to have immediate families that are overweight. However, all of their great-great-grandparents were almost certainly of normal weight. If their ancestors could be lean with identical genetic material, the cause of their weight gain must be in their current environment. It must be something to which only certain people are susceptible, just as some of us can have a fatal allergic reaction to a small amount of peanuts, while others can't eat enough.[1] Genes protect some of us, but not most of us, from being affected.

While genes are a major enabler of weight gain, genetic change cannot be the cause. Up until the beginning of the 20th century, less than 1% of Americans were severely overweight. Today that number is closer to 34%. There is no theory which suggests how the human genome could evolve rapidly enough to account for such a major change in the population. Furthermore, for evolution to be a cause of the increase, being overweight would need to give some type of evolutionary advantage. In fact, this is not the case. Being overweight is associated with health problems including decreased fertility.[2]

---

[1] Powell, Alvin. "Obesity runs in families - and friends, too." Harvard University Gazette. 4/04/2009 <http://www.news.harvard.edu/gazette/2007/03.08/09-obesity.html>.
[2] Lucas, Michael. "Obesity may decrease men's fertility, a new study suggests." HeatlhHype.com. 4/04/2009 <http://www.healthhype.com/obesity-may-decrease-men%E2%80%99s-fertility-a-new-study-suggests.html>.

The Real Role of Genetics in Weight Gain

Human genetics cannot explain the over 3,000% increase in the number of Americans who have become severely overweight since the beginning of the 20th century, but they may be able to explain why scientists have had such a hard time identifying the real culprit. To study what causes weight gain, scientists want to look at the actions of a group of people over time, see who gained weight, and figure out what they did differently from those who did not gain weight. But what if some people in our group are not going to gain much weight no matter what they do because of a genetic variation they have? To complicate matters, what if that genetic variation occurs at different rates in different countries?

The genetic disparity in the way various groups react to specific factors in their diet takes away one of the most useful tools researchers have. The Western diet is associated with weight gain wherever it becomes more prevalent. When immigrants from low weight countries move to the U.S., those who keep their traditional diets remain lean, while many of those who adopt the American diet gain weight.

The components of the Western diet include refined grains, sugars, red meat, vegetable oils, dairy products, coffee, and soft drinks. Since scientists know that this diet is associated with weight gain, one of the first things they try to do when studying the obesity level of a country's population is to examine its consumption of each of these parts of the diet, in order to try to figure out which cause weight gain. However, this approach does not work. For each of these components, there are countries where consumption is very high but people are very thin. The same is true of different groups within the United States. We all know people who "can't get fat." This observation has scientific backing. Estimates for the importance of genetics in predicting obesity in the United States have ranged as high as 85%.

Because we are in only the very early stage of understanding the effects of our genetic variations, scientists are unable to genetically screen out from their studies the people who cannot easily become overweight. If we could do such screening, it would be relatively easy to look at the differences in diet between lean people and those who have become overweight, without the confusion caused by any genetic factors that keep people thin despite their diet.

Studies of identical twins can eliminate genes as a factor in obesity, but they have been performed to only a small degree. It is not easy to follow large numbers of twins for a long enough period of time to be able to see differences in their diets and diet outcomes. It is easier to try to understand the mechanism causing genetically predisposed people to become overweight. For the data we have, comparisons are going to help us only when we look at the same country over time.[1]

In addition to confounding scientists, the idea that genes, by themselves, cause weight gain has done a lot of damage to individuals. If you think your weight problems are genetic, that is akin to saying that they are beyond your control, and it can stop

[1] Yang, Wenjie . "Genetic Epidemiology of Obesity." Epidemiologic Reviews. 4/04/2009 <http://epirev.oxfordjournals.org/cgi/content/abstract/29/1/49>.

you from believing that it is in your power to find a solution. Even if you are overweight, barring a rare genetic disease that you would probably be aware you had, all of your ancestors were extremely lean until about a hundred years ago. There is a set of circumstances that will make you thin as well.

Over the last 150 years, there have been enormous changes in our environment. A large number of us have become overweight in response to these changes, but many of us have genes that have protected us from gaining weight. Since people have never before lived in a period in which weight gain has been widespread, these genes must have developed for another reason, and they must have some other function. After all, we can't develop a new gene and spread it to a large part of the human race in a hundred years, so any such gene which exists would have to also perform another function. Scientists have not yet established with certainty what the function is, but we will see a possible explanation later.

Ethnicity and Weight Gain

One identifiable genetic trait that corresponds to our ability to gain weight is ethnicity. After adjusting for income level, education, and diet, there are still variations among ethnic groups in the United States that can be explained only by genetic differences.[1]

Comparing residents of Japan and Japanese Americans allows us to observe this relationship. According to the 2008 *Central Intelligence Agency World Factbook*, Japan's populace has the longest life expectancy of any major country. Only Andorra, with a population of 70,000, has a slightly higher life expectancy. Japanese born today are expected to live 82 years, compared to 78 years for people born in the United States today. In addition, the Japanese have the lowest rate of people in the developed world who are severely overweight, at about 3% in 2005, according to the *Organization for Economic Cooperation and Development Factbook*. This was over 90% less than in the United States in the same year.

One explanation for this could be that genetics are largely or entirely responsible. The Japanese and American populations are ethnically different, and all of the East Asian countries have lower rates of obesity than ethnically European countries. There is an easy way to test if this is true, and that is to look at Japanese immigrants to the United States. What we find is that as Japanese immigrants adopt the American diet, they tend to gain weight. In fact, even in Japan, people are gaining weight as Western food becomes more prevalent. However, the Japanese in Japan and

---

[1]Fernández, José R. "Using Genetic Admixture to Study the Biology of Obesity Traits and to Map Genes in Admixed Populations." Nutrition Reviews. 4/03/2009 <http://www3.interscience.wiley.com/journal/120843214/abstract?CRETRY=1&SRETRY=0>.

Japanese immigrants in the United States remain thinner than many other ethnic groups.[1]

This tells us that, even if genes are partially responsible, there is something in the American diet which is not so prevalent in the Japanese diet which causes weight gain in people who have that genetic predisposition. If we can identify this substance and remove it, we should be able to eliminate the modern problem of obesity. Since obesity has been linked to an assortment of chronic health problems, we may even start to live as long as the Japanese.

---

[1] Kovacs, Jenny. "Diets of the World: The Japanese Diet." WebMD. 4/04/2009 <http://www.webmd.com/diet/features/diets-of-world-japanese-diet>.

Calories and Weight Gain

The United States Food and Drug Administration (FDA) is the government agency charged with "assuring the safety, efficacy, and security of human and veterinary drugs . . . our nation's food supply . . . [It] is also responsible for . . . helping the public get the accurate, science-based information they need to use medicines and foods to improve their health."[1] That includes giving Americans the information they need to stay thin.

The FDA is very aware that Americans are getting fatter. As part of its efforts to combat the problem, the agency is planning to "[work] to help consumers make smart choices about their diet." How will the FDA do this? Actions the FDA wants to take include "strengthening food labeling, . . . educating consumers about maintaining a healthy diet and weight, and encouraging restaurants to provide calorie and nutrition information."[2]

Endorsed By the Experts

The FDA also wants to "increase enforcement to ensure food labels accurately portray serving size and strengthen scientific research aimed at . . . developing foods that are healthier and lower in calories." According to an article by Linda Bren titled "Losing Weight—Start By Counting Calories" published in the

---

[1] "FDA's Mission Statement." FDA. 4/04/2009 <http://www.fda.gov/opacom/morechoices/mission.html>.

[2] Bren, Linda. "Losing Weight: Start By Counting Calories." FDA. 4/04/2009 <http://www.fda.gov/FDAC/features/2002/102_fat.html>.

FDA Consumer magazine, "the experts . . . generally agree that the key to losing weight is a simple message: Eat less and move more. Your body needs to burn more calories than you take in."[1]

Also in the article on losing weight are some tips to staying thin for people who are dining out. They include:

> Ask for nutrition information (for example, calories, saturated fat, and sodium) before you order when eating out. Choose foods that are steamed, broiled, baked, roasted, poached, or stir-fried, but not deep-fat fried. Share food, such as a main dish or dessert, with your dining partner. Take part of the food home with you and refrigerate immediately. You may want to ask for a take-home container when the meal arrives. Spoon half the meal into it, so you're more likely to eat only what's left on your plate. Request your meal to be served without gravy, sauces, butter or margarine. Ask for salad dressing on the side, and use only small amounts of full-fat dressings.[2]

The FDA's statements can be assumed to reflect consensus opinions of the American medical establishment; it is a very mainstream organization. As we read the above tips on weight loss, we see that the FDA implicates too much fat and too many calories as being responsible for weight gain. There are really no other possible dietary culprits mentioned.

---

[1] Idem.
[2] Idem.

The FDA also suggests that we need to make sure we are eating the right sizes of portions and that we need to not eat too much at restaurants. It advises, "Share food . . . with [a] partner." In this report, the FDA clearly demonstrates the belief that we are simply choosing to overeat because we are undisciplined, and fat is partially to blame. However, we have seen previously that eating too much fat is not responsible for weight gain. If it were, then the Inuit who left their traditional high fat diet for a relatively lower fat Western diet would not have gained weight while those Inuit who stayed with their traditional diet remained thin.

Furthermore, if too much fat caused weight gain, those people who adopted the high fat Atkins diet would have gained large amounts of weight, but they did not. We have many examples of people staying thin on a high fat diet and gaining weight on a low fat diet. Thus, we can see that this FDA report is incorrect in placing the blame for weight gain on fat consumption. What about eating too many calories and not exercising enough? This FDA article was published before the government study which found that diet and exercise were no more beneficial than diet alone was published. So if lack of exercise isn't responsible for obesity, is eating too many calories the culprit? Perhaps we are simply choosing to eat too much.

Counting Calories

Counting calories is an idea that became popular around the beginning of the 20th century, probably because this was the beginning of the period of modern weight gain. At that time, a scientist noticed that, if food was burned in a machine, the amount of heat it produced could be measured to find out how much chemical energy was released. From this, it was possible to figure out how much energy was in the food. The calorie is the unit used to measure this food energy. The idea that the cause of becoming overweight is eating too many calories has become more and more popular. Many diet books were written early in the 20th century, claiming that it is "all about calories," and the idea has become more entrenched since.

It is this idea that has led to laws requiring that all packaged foods in the United States be labeled with how many calories they contain, as well as how many grams of protein, fat, and carbohydrates. It is this idea, in part, which has led to the idea that we should eat less fat, since fat is calorically dense; by eating less fat we could eat bulkier food that would make us feel fuller but contain fewer calories. However, this begs the question: Counting calories is an idea that has been around for almost a hundred years. During that period, Americans have become more and more overweight. That seems to imply that it isn't really "all about the calories."[1]

This is not to say the idea of calories has no meaning. One pound of human fat stores 3,500 calories. Expend 3,500 more calories than you take in, and your body has to get that energy either by breaking down your fat reserves or by taking it from other body tissues such as your muscles. Therefore, if being overweight is just "all about the calories," someone who is overweight is just a person who has eaten too much for the

---

[1] Kovacs, Jenny Stamos . "The Dos and Don'ts of Counting Calories." WebMD. 4/04/2009 <http://www.webmd.com/diet/features/dos-donts-counting-calories>.

amount of energy he has used. Take enough food away from that person, and he or she should be just the same as a person of normal weight.[1]

Body Weight Regulation

We do not have to imagine what would happen if we took calories away from an overweight person. It is an experiment that has been done in laboratories many times. Overweight people have been put on very-low-calorie liquid diets. They have lost lots of weight, but too much lean body mass and not enough fat. Still, it is not uncommon for people to lose 15 to 20 pounds of fat on a liquid diet and have a massive fall in their cholesterol levels. Unfortunately, what is also not uncommon and, in fact, seems to happen in the majority of cases, is that all of the weight lost and even more is gained back within three years.[2]

The reasons are not psychological: The people in these experiments are not simply making a decision to eat too much. People who are overweight but lose a lot of fat are not like people who were never overweight in the first place. They are like normal people who are in near-starvation mode. The metabolism of people in one study dropped from normal to burning 24% fewer calories per day. They dreamt of food and of leaving the diet. They became anxious and depressed, if not suicidal. They

---

[1] "Counting calories: Getting back to weight-loss basics." Mayo Clinic. 4/04/2009 <http://www.mayoclinic.com/health/calories/WT00011>.

[2] Burros, Marian. "Diet Formulas: Losing the Weight Is the Easy Part." New York Times. 4/11/2009 <http://www.nytimes.com/1988/07/06/garden/diet-formulas-losing-the-weight-is-the-easy-part.html>.

hid food in their rooms. When they left the program, they ate massive amounts of food. The few who did not regain the weight they had lost were always hungry and had to constantly resist the urge to eat.

This leads to the question of whether it is possible that once a person gains weight he or she can never return to being of normal weight. Another study proved this idea wrong as well. Dr. Ethan Sims of the University of Vermont wanted to know what would happen if anyone who had never had a weight problem became fat. Would the person have a lifelong problem and never be able to return to a normal weight? To find out, he got volunteers from a state prison who agreed to try and gain weight. They were successful, and over a period of four to six months, eating as much as they could every day, they increased their weight by 20 to 25 percent. Everything they ate was recorded, and some even ate 10,000 calories a day.[1]

However, unlike the overweight people who had normal metabolic levels, these people who had become fat intentionally had metabolisms that rose to 50% above normal. They had no problem returning to their normal weight. After the study, it took them a few months to return to their pre-experiment level and stay there. This was not because prison food was making them thin, as about 23% of prisoners in the United States are obese.[2]

---

[1] Kolata, Gina. "Genes Take Charge, and Diets Fall by the Wayside." New York Times. 4/04/2009 <http://www.nytimes.com/2007/05/08/health/08fat.html?_r=3&oref=slogin>.
[2] Houle, Brian. "Obesity prevalence among male inmates and how their inclusion affects race-education disparities in U.S. national obesity prevalence." Princeton University. 4/04/2009 <http://paa2009.princeton.edu/download.aspx?submissionId=90951>.

This seems to challenge the FDA's theory that Americans are simply overeating. After all, if we were, it would be just as easy for us to return to a normal weight as it was for the volunteers in this study. Clearly, the government's weight loss plan is in error.

We can learn from this study what the author intended, that becoming overweight does not doom someone to staying that way his entire life. However, that is not the only thing we can learn. The study shows that the body has powerful and not fully understood mechanisms for regulating our weight. For most of human history, that mechanism has maintained our weight with slight variation. If we did not have enough food, we would become hungrier and our metabolism would fall. If we had too much food, our metabolism would rise and we would feel full.

When our bodies work as they should, we are able to maintain a relatively constant weight, even if caloric intake varies from day to day. Our body has a mechanism to deal with overeating; it raises metabolism and it increases feelings of fullness. This results in weight being lost easily. The problem for those of us who are overweight is not that we have eaten too many calories. The real problem for those of us who need to lose weight is that our body's weight regulatory mechanism is not working properly.

We are born without knowing language or anything else about the world, yet even as babies we know when we are hungry and we get very upset when we are not fed. As babies, our bodies seem to unconsciously know how much to eat. After all, despite not consciously knowing anything, babies will not fail to cry if they have not been fed or to stop eating when they have had enough. So either we have lost this mechanism as adults or something is interfering with it. To lose weight, what we need to do is identify the substance that is keeping this mechanism from working properly.

Unconventional Obesity Theories

Much of the public still accepts the ideas that genetics, carbohydrates, fats, or a sedentary lifestyle can explain the obesity epidemic. On the other hand, many obesity researchers have realized that traditional theories do not explain what we are witnessing in the modern era, and they have come up with some unconventional theories. In 2006 the *International Journal of Obesity* published an article titled "Putative contributors to the secular increase in obesity: exploring the roads less traveled."[1] The article was a list of highly unconventional theories for the causes of increasing levels of obesity. After a CBS News report, the list gained some prominence and is popular on many internet message boards. Here are a few that we have not addressed.

Pollution

Theory: The increase in the rate of obesity has corresponded with an increase in industrial pollution. Many of these pollutants are known as endocrine disruptors, chemicals that can interfere with hormones in our bodies. Hormones regulate appetite, and appetite controls body weight. Thus, a chemical that interferes with our hormones could make us overweight.

Fact: There are examples of drugs that can cause weight gain by interfering with our hormones; however, if pollution were

---

[1] Keith, S. "Putative contributors to the secular increase in obesity: exploring the roads less traveled." International Journal of Obesity. 4/04/2009 <http://www.nature.com/ijo/journal/v30/n11/abs/0803326a.html>.

the cause of obesity, then people in very different countries would be overweight. For example, Japan is arguably almost as technologically advanced as the United States and is much more urban, with people more exposed to the pollution city life brings. In Beijing, China, air pollution is so bad that athletes at the 2008 Olympic Games brought facemasks.[1] It is not unusual for facemasks to be worn in Japanese and Chinese cities. Yet both these countries have obesity rates that are more than 90% lower than in the United States. Since the United States has lower pollution levels than Japan, but Japanese who move to the United States gain weight, pollution does not appear to explain increasing obesity.

Air Conditioning

Theory: The number of people in the United States who have air conditioning has also increased at the same time as the rates of obesity. Since we have to burn calories to heat or cool our bodies, air conditioning should cause a fall in the amount of calories we burn. This decrease could lead to an increase in weight.

Fact: This also does not fit with the examples of France and Japan, where air conditioning is just as common as in the United States. Air conditioning is simply another factor that correlates with our increased wealth. It also does not explain why Japanese

[1] "Japan Olympians Pack Face Masks for Beijing." Javno. 4/04/2009 <http://www.javno.com/en-sports/japan-olympians-pack-face-masks-for-beijing_167699>.

immigrants to the United States who keep their traditional diets remain thin, while those who adopt the Western diet gain weight.

Decreased Smoking

Theory: Nicotine is a drug, and one of the effects of nicotine on our bodies is to lower our appetite. Since the discovery that smoking causes lung cancer, a major campaign has been conducted to get Americans to smoke less. This effort has resulted in a decrease in the rate of Americans who smoke, and this could cause an increase in the number of overweight people.

Fact: Tobacco has been used in the Americas since before they were discovered by Europeans. It wasn't introduced to Europe until after the discovery. Still, for thousands of years Europeans were quite lean without the use of tobacco, so decreased smoking seems an unlikely candidate for the cause of the increased rates of obesity in Europe or America. It especially cannot explain the rise of childhood obesity. After all, how could childhood obesity formerly have been prevented by smoking when the number of children smoking was insignificant?

Older Moms

Theory: Another proposed theory is that the increase in obesity can be tied to the higher rate of women who are giving birth at later ages. There is a correlation between the age of a woman at birth and the probability her children will be overweight.

Fact: There is also a correlation between age and wealth. Women who give birth when they are older have higher incomes, on average. This means they are more likely to eat out at restaurants. Eating meals at restaurants is also correlated with weight gain.

A Fat-Causing Virus

Theory: Of all the unusual suggestions for the cause of obesity, my personal favorite is a fat-causing virus. We are gaining weight because of a new disease that is making us fat.

Fact: Recall that Japanese in the U.S. who still eat their traditional diet remain much thinner than those who adopt the American diet. For a virus to be the cause of increasing obesity levels, it would have to be able to distinguish between these two groups, and that seems somewhat unlikely.

Eliminating the Impossible

All of these theories seem to be incorrect, but all of them are excellent science. Trial and error are an integral part of the process of discovery. Thomas Edison, who invented the first practical electric light bulb and was one of the most prolific inventors who ever lived, spent a year and a half testing hundreds of different substances before discovering the carbon filament.

Rather than viewing his early tests as failures, he saw them as discovering what would not work. They were clues on the path to finding the one right material. In Edison's day, the idea that an electric light could be used to illuminate homes probably seemed just as unlikely as the idea that a virus is responsible for weight gain today. In that respect we can still learn from Edison, who said that discovery, "is about turning a wild goose chase into a fox hunt."[1] Once we eliminate what does not work, what is left is what does. Knowing that all of these theories cannot explain weight gain frees us to look for new theories.

---

[1] "Edisonian approach." Wikipedia. 4/04/2009 <http://en.wikipedia.org/wiki/Edisonian_approach>.

Part II: Current Weight Loss Research

"Everyone hears only what he understands."
-Johann Wolfgang von Goethe

If we want to lose weight, we are faced with a scientific question, even if we do not think of it that way. We have to answer the question, "What causes weight gain?" We have to answer that question because we are bombarded with many different diets that claim to be the best way to lose weight. Since most of us are getting fatter rather than thinner, we can assume the majority of these methods do not work. We need to be detectives in order to find what really is effective. Since we have already ruled out many ideas that are incorrect, we will not fall into the trap of using failed ideas to understand unexplained weight loss research. This is important, because most weight loss research is not satisfactorily explained, or we would all be thin.

There are many scientists who are trying to answer the mystery of modern weight gain. Thousands of doctors and researchers have dedicated their lives to trying to solve this problem. By looking at some of the interesting things they have discovered, we may find clues that can help us narrow down the possible causes of weight gain. Researchers have already discovered many things that happen with weight gain—things that people who gain weight tend to do or experience. Scientists have also discovered some things that even predict weight gain.

What is left for us to do is piece together the puzzle of why all these things occur together. For example, why is it that soda causes weight gain? It doesn't sound surprising, until you learn that people who drink diet soda are even more likely to become overweight than people who drink regular soda. How does this fit in with the fact that overweight people are hungrier than thinner people, tend to sleep less, and experience higher levels of stress?

Facts like these are a puzzle, and the first step in solving a puzzle is looking at all of the pieces. Once we can solve these unanswered questions in weight loss research, we will have the true reason for the cause of modern weight gain. With that, we should be able to return to being as thin as our ancestors were for thousands of years. So let us look at the first piece of our puzzle.

Soda and Weight Gain

Recent studies have demonstrated that soda consumption is a risk factor for weight gain. This does not surprise people, because conventional wisdom holds that sugar causes weight gain. Since most soda is filled with sugar, this theory would predict that soda would cause weight gain. However, what it would not predict is that diet soda, which contains almost no calories, would also cause weight gain. In fact, diet soda consumption is an even stronger predictor of weight gain than is consumption of regular soda. In an eight-year study of 1,500 Americans at the University of Texas Health Science Center, 622 started at a normal weight. About one-third of these 622 participants became obese or overweight over the course of the study, and the amount of soda they drank was a strong predictor of whether they would become overweight. Here are the percentages of the normal weight participants who became overweight or obese, according to their soda consumption:[1]

Consumption	Regular Soda	Diet Soda
up to 1/2 can daily	26.0%	36.5%
1/2 to 1 can daily	30.4%	37.5%
1 to 2 cans daily	32.8%	54.5%
over 2 cans daily	47.2%	57.1%

[1] DeNoon, Daniel J. "Drink More Diet Soda, Gain More Weight?" WebMD. 4/04/2009 <http://www.webmd.com/diet/news/20050613/drink-more-diet-soda-gain-more-weight>.

To most people, the mystery here is why diet soda causes weight gain, while they readily accept that soda made with sugar, a carbohydrate, causes weight gain. Remember, we have already seen that sugar in 100% fruit juice does not cause weight gain. People have been cultivating fruit and making fruit juices for thousands of years. People on the Atkins diet who give up almost all sugar do not experience long-term weight loss.

Of course, this does not necessarily mean that soda causes weight gain. Perhaps people who eat fast food are more likely to drink soda, and something in fast food causes weight gain. This would explain why soda consumption seems to cause weight gain, but it would not explain why diet soda is about 36% more likely to be associated with weight gain than is regular soda.

We are trying to solve a mystery here, and we have to look at every theory no matter how improbable, so let us see if diet soda can be responsible for the increasing levels of obesity since the start of the 20th century. The answer, of course, is a resounding, "No," because the first diet soda was introduced to the United States in 1982, long after the obesity epidemic was underway. This means that, even if diet soda has contributed to increased obesity, it does not explain the weight gain seen over the prior 80 years. Then there is the theory that artificial sweeteners, which became popular in the 1950s, cause weight gain, but this does not explain why regular soda causes weight gain. Why should sugar in regular soda cause weight gain when the sugar in 100% fruit juice does not?

Sleep Deprivation and Weight Gain

As a society, we began going to sleep later almost as soon as the invention of the electric light in the 19th century. Children are instinctively afraid of the dark, and in modern times many children have small "night lights" in their rooms, to help quell this innate fear. However, it was not so long ago that adults feared the dark as well.

The ancient walled cities of the Fertile Crescent, such as Jerusalem, Babylon, Jericho, and Uruk, all closed at sunset. Travelers feared having to make camp outside the city walls, where they were easy prey for bandits. For all of our history, until late in the 19th century, most people stayed home after sunset, with only the light of a fire or oil lamp to keep them awake. Due to the availability of artificial lighting alone, it should not be surprising that we are sleeping less. It simply does not occur to us to be home by sunset any more, whereas a hundred years ago there may have been nothing but moonlight to guide us outside.

There have been several studies that suggest that people who are sleep-deprived are much more likely to gain weight.[1,2] As a result of significant scientific studies like these, which have identified what appears to be a valid correlation between sleeping

---

[1] "Sleep Deprivation Doubles Risks Of Obesity In Both Children And Adults." Science Daily. 4/04/2009 <http://www.sciencedaily.com/releases/2006/07/060713081140.htm>.
[2] Weaver, Nicole. "Sleep Deprivation Plays Role in Obesity." Daily News Central. 4/04/2009 <http://health.dailynewscentral.com/content/view/2594/>.

less and gaining weight, erroneous articles have been published suggesting the key to losing weight may be just to try to sleep more.[1]

Leading to More Confusion

It is no wonder so many people give up hope on dieting. So much information is presented in a way that is unhelpful to most people. While these studies have taught us something valuable, it is not that trying to sleep more will make us thin. After all, perhaps gaining weight makes us sleep less? Maybe not exercising enough makes it difficult to sleep and causes weight gain (although I am not suggesting this).

In reality, people who are overweight are diagnosed with sleep disorders more often than are people of normal weight.[2] Knowing that the odds of weight gain are greater among people who do not get enough sleep is very important to weight researchers, because it tells them that whatever is causing people to gain weight may also be causing them to lose sleep. This tends to point the blame away from things like eating fats, sugars, and refined carbohydrates and towards things like drinking caffeine, which is associated with not being able to sleep enough.

---

[1] Stein, Rob. "Scientists Finding Out What Losing Sleep Does to a Body." Washington Post. 4/04/2009 <http://www.washingtonpost.com/wp-dyn/content/article/2005/10/08/AR2005100801405.html>.
[2] Stacy, Kelli. "Obesity Ups Odds of Short Sleep." MedicineNet.com. 4/04/2009 <http://www.medicinenet.com/script/main/art.asp?articlekey=89201>.

Caffeine and Sleep

Caffeine can cause measurable disturbances to sleep after taking as little as 200 milligrams (mg), about the weight of an adult size aspirin. This is less caffeine than what is in the average large soda in a casual dining restaurant, and it is less than the average amount consumed daily by the typical American. Higher amounts of caffeine consumption can cause severe problems. The *Diagnostic and Statistical Manual of Mental Disorders* (DSM), the main book used to classify mental diseases, lists "caffeine-induced sleep disorder" as a psychiatric disorder.[1]

Unable to Sleep or Choosing not to Sleep

We can set an alarm clock and wake ourselves up early, but the need for sleep catches up with us. Eventually, we have to make up the lost time. Rather than blaming weight gain on not sleeping enough, we would be better off examining factors that are correlated with insufficient sleep. These include caffeine, but they could also include exercise, sunlight exposure, and other drugs. The theory of this book is not that people gain weight because they do not sleep enough. Instead, it presents the theory

[1] Huetteman, John . "The link between caffeine consumption and sleep disorders." Helium. 4/04/2009 <http://www.helium.com/items/475985-the-link-between-caffeine-consumption-and-sleep-disorders>.

that whatever is causing people to gain weight is also causing them to sleep less.[1]

[1] Sobel, David. " Exercise Improves Sleep." Health World. 4/04/2009 <http://www.healthy.net/scr/article.asp?ID=424>.

The Hunger-Obesity Paradox

It is popularly assumed that people who are overweight have eaten too much or have eaten "bad" or "fattening" foods. Many psychological reasons are given for why people do this, such as boredom, laziness, and the abundance of food. However, while people who are overweight have eaten too much, there is evidence that their reasons for doing so are physiological rather than psychological.

Hunger with Overeating

Though it is counterintuitive, or contrary to the way we naturally think, people who have gained weight by eating too much are likely to be hungrier than those who have not. Since eating usually causes us to feel full, and not eating causes us to be hungry, why overweight people are hungrier than thin people has been a mystery. It has been called the Hunger-Obesity Paradox by health researchers.[1]

The popular explanation for this paradox among researchers is that it is caused by food insecurity. The theory goes that it is poor people who are most likely to be overweight, and people who are poor are more likely to be fearful about their future

---

[1]Harrison, Gail. "The Paradox of Hunger and Obesity." California Center for Population Research. 4/04/2009 <http://repositories.cdlib.org/cgi/viewcontent.cgi?article=1190&context=ccpr>.

ability to feed themselves. This stress then causes food-insecure people to overeat.

There are many problems with this explanation for the hunger-obesity paradox. While poor people in the United States are more likely to be overweight,[1] in China it is rich people who are more likely to be overweight.[2] This seems to rule out food-insecurity as a cause of the hunger-obesity paradox.

An Important Clue

Thus, we are left with a very important paradox, without a conventional explanation. However, this paradox points to the mechanism responsible for the obesity epidemic. As a society, we are gaining weight because we are hungrier. When we look for the cause of weight gain and for what might cause weight loss, we need to look for things that will have an effect on our hunger.

This is a major departure from traditional dieting and medical advice. Indeed, you cannot buy packaged food at a supermarket in the United States without the amount of calories being displayed on the packaging. At the same time, we have

---

[1]Harrison, Gail. "The Paradox of Hunger and Obesity." California Center for Population Research. 4/04/2009
<http://repositories.cdlib.org/cgi/viewcontent.cgi?article=1190&context=ccpr>.
[2]"China: Affluence Brings Obesity." New York Times. 4/04/2009
<http://query.nytimes.com/gst/fullpage.html?res=9905EFD7113FF934A35752C1A9609C8B63>.

almost no awareness of what will make us hungrier, and we have collectively become much hungrier.

Eating More

In the U.S., both the amount of food produced per person and the amount of food eaten per person have dramatically increased in recent history. In 1978, we were producing 3,200 calories of food per person. By 1999, the food industry was producing 3,900 calories of food per person.[1] Adjusting for a higher amount of waste, over two decades we increased food consumption by 418 calories per person.

This explains the average increase of Americans' weight over the same period. It is not that we are eating more simply because more food is available. After all, food is subject to the same economic laws of supply and demand as any other product. If farmers produced more food than was being demanded, they would create a surplus. A surplus would cause prices to drop and lower the incentive to produce food. This would cause production to fall until a new equilibrium was reached.

This extra food is being demanded and consumed. What we see in these facts is the effect of the Hunger-Obesity paradox on the national level. Americans are eating more because they are

---

[1] David M.. "Why Have Americans Become More Obese?" Economic Research Service. 4/04/2009 <http://www.ers.usda.gov/publications/efan04004/efan04004b.pdf>.

hungrier, and they are hungrier despite eating enough to gain substantial amounts of weight.

What is needed to solve the problem of weight gain is not a way to will ourselves to eat less. What is needed is to identify the cause or causes of the increased hunger we are experiencing in the modern age in the United States and Europe. Some of these causes are, in fact, known and studied, but they are usually ignored in popular books on diet. One of the few exceptions to this is a book called *The Shangri-La Diet*.[1] In the next chapter, we will look at substances that are known to cause weight gain. Such weight gain is not occurring because of a change in metabolism. We are consuming substances that cause an increase in hunger, which leads to increased eating and, eventually, substantial weight gain.

---

[1] Roberts, Dr. Seth. *The Shangri-La Diet: The No Hunger Eat Anything Weight-Loss Plan.* Perigee, 2007.

Prescription Drugs and Weight Gain

This section is about the existence of drugs that can cause weight gain by increasing hunger. It is not a call for us to abandon prescription drugs. In the United States, the average person born at the beginning of the 20th century could expect to live to about age 47. By 2008, despite increased obesity, life expectancy at birth had risen to about 78.[1]

Most deaths at the beginning of the 20th century were from infectious disease. Today in the United States, infectious disease isn't even in the top three causes of death. The top two causes are now heart disease and stroke, for which being overweight is a major risk factor.[2]

Fortunately, while weight gain can be a side effect of many prescription drugs for some people, different drugs cause weight gain in different people. If a prescription drug can be identified as a cause of weight gain, it may be possible for you and your doctor to try alternative drugs. For those of us who are not taking any of these drugs, the following list is still interesting, because it shows us how common it is for drugs to cause weight gain by affecting appetite. It is not always understood why they have this effect,

---

[1] "CIA – The World Factbook – Field Listing - Life expectancy at birth." Central Intelligence Agency. 4/04/2009 <https://www.cia.gov/library/publications/the-world-factbook/fields/2102.html>.

[2] Mauk, Kristen. *Gerontological Nursing: Competencies for Care.* Jones & Bartlett Publishers, 2006.

but none of these drugs has been shown to cause weight gain by altering metabolism. This list is just a sample.

Drugs with Weight Gain as a Side Effect

Class:	Anticonvulsants
Names:	Lamictal, Tegretol
Effects:	Used mainly to treat seizure disorders but also prescribed to treat bipolar disorder and certain types of depression.
Appetite:	Anticonvulsants tend to cause elevated insulin levels in the blood (hyperinsulinemia) and increased appetite. Increased appetite leads to weight gain.[1]

Class:	Antidepressants
Names:	Paxil, Zoloft, Prozac
Effects:	Used to treat major depression. The exact mechanism of the therapeutic effects is controversial.
Appetite:	The specific mechanism is unknown, but it is known that antidepressants are associated with increased food cravings and an inability to feel full despite eating more than enough.[2]

---

[1] Riley, Gay. "The Relationship between Weight Gain and Medications for Depression and Seizures." NetNutritionist.com. 4/04/2009 <http://www.netnutritionist.com/fa12.htm>.
[2] Ruetsch, Viala. "Psychotropic drugs induced weight gain." The Good Drug Guide. 4/04/2009 <http://biopsychiatry.com/weight-gain.htm>.

Class:	Antipsychotics
Names:	Zyprexa, Seroquel, Risperdal
Effects:	Used to treat schizophrenia, mania, delusional disorder, and psychotic depression. They work by blocking receptors in the brain's dopamine pathways.
Appetite:	Animal studies have suggested that antipsychotics affect appetite regulation.[1]

Class:	Beta-Blockers
Names:	Tenormin, Lopressor
Effects:	Used in the treatment of high blood pressure, panic attacks, and abnormal heart rhythms. Block adrenalin, causing heart rate to slow.
Appetite:	The older Beta-Blockers caused high blood insulin level, which is associated with increased hunger. The newer Beta-Blockers are not associated with weight gain.[2]

Class:	Mood Stabilizers
Names:	Lithium, Depakote, Seroquel
Effects:	Used to treat mood disorders in which there are intense and persistent mood shifts, including bipolar disorder. Also used to treat borderline (psychotic) personality disorder.

---

[1] "Antipsychotic medications: Is weight gain inevitable?" Mayo Clinic. 4/04/2009 <http://www.mayoclinic.com/health/antipsychotic-medications/AN01685>.
[2] Mirkin, Gabe. "Beta Blockers Side Effects" www.DrMirkin.com . 4/04/2009 <http://www.drmirkin.com/heart/7642.html>.

Appetite:	Cause increased appetite and cravings for sweet and fatty foods.[1]

Class:	Steroids
Names:	Prednisone, Triamcinolone, Betamethasone
Effects:	Steroids, which are different from anabolic-steroids used by weight builders to gain muscle, are used to treat inflammatory conditions such as dermatitis, arthritis, and asthma.
Appetite:	Steroids cause weight gain in nearly all patients who take them.[2]

Class:	Antihistamines
Names:	Allegra, Benadryl, Zyrtec
Effect:	Used as treatment for allergies. They inhibit the release of histamine, which is released in excessive amounts in people with allergies.
Appetite:	May increase hunger because histamine receptors are involved in appetite regulation. While people do not complain that they feel hungry, it is observed that they are eating more.[3] Occurs in a small percentage of patients.

Class:	Non-Steroidal Anti-Inflammatories (NSAIDS)

---

[1] Ruetsch, Viala. "Psychotropic drugs induced weight gain." The Good Drug Guide. 4/04/2009 <http://biopsychiatry.com/weight-gain.htm>.

[2] "Prednisone Information." Johns Hopkins Vasculitis Center. 4/04/2009 <http://vasculitis.med.jhu.edu/treatments/prednisone.html#weight>.

[3] Duenwalkd, Mary. "Is Your Medicine Cabinet Making You Fat? " New York Times. 4/04/2009 <http://www.nytimes.com/2005/08/16/health/16cons.html>.

Names:	Celecoxib, Nimesulide, Licofelone
Effect:	Used as treatment for pain and inflammation in conditions such as headache, migraine, arthritis, and gout. They inhibit the action of the enzyme cyclooxygenase.
Appetite:	Weight gain is a reported side effect of NSAIDS but the mechanism of action has not been studied.[1]

[1]"Medication Guide for Non-Steroidal Anti-Inflammatory Drugs." FDA. 4/04/2009 <http://www.fda.gov/CDER/drug/infopage/COX2/NSAIDmedguide.htm>.

Cortisol, Stress, and Weight Gain

When we think of stress, we often think of it as an emotion, what we feel when we cannot cope with what life throws at us. We think of stress as something that exists in our heads separate from our bodies, but this is not all that stress is. While we may experience stress as an emotion, our body experiences stress physically. During periods of stress and anxiety our adrenal glands produce a "fight or flight" hormone called cortisol.

Cortisol Is the Stress Hormone

This hormone is not just a result of the feeling of stress; it causes the feeling of stress. Scientists have determined this by raising the level of cortisol in mice and observing their behavior. They have found that the mice experienced symptoms of anxiety and lowered reactions to outside stimuli. This is a sign of their nervous systems being overwhelmed and is typical of stress in humans.[1]

Cortisol affects our entire body. It increases blood pressure and blood sugar, reduces the action of the immune system, slows bone formation, and more. All of these reactions might help us if we needed to escape from an attack or fend off a pack of

---

[1]Dombeck, Mark. "Chronic cortisol exposure causes mood disorders." MentalHelp.net. 4/04/2009
<http://www.mentalhelp.net/poc/view_doc.php?type=weblog&id=68&wlid=6&cn=5>.

predators, but they are of much less use to us today than when they originated.

Because of cortisol, chronic stress is associated with a wide range of health conditions. Chronic stress and chronically high cortisol levels can lower the body's ability to resist infection. Stress is also thought to be the cause of many skin conditions, back pain, stomachaches, diarrhea, and, most interestingly for us, weight gain.

Stress and Weight Gain

Soon after we get into a stressful situation, one of the things we usually want to do is eat. Imagine someone suddenly cuts you off in traffic and you have to brake immediately to avoid an accident. Your heart beats a little bit faster, you breathe a little bit more heavily, you feel angry, but you don't necessarily feel hungry immediately. This is because you have just released adrenaline, and adrenaline is an amphetamine. Like all amphetamines, in addition to making you awake and alert, it reduces your hunger.[1]

As a result of a stressful situation, your blood cortisol level also increases, and it stays elevated longer than your adrenaline level. Cortisol acts to help you recover from the effects of the

---

[1] "Educating Students about Drug Use and Mental Health." Centre for Addiction and Mental Health. 4/04/2009 <http://www.camh.net/education/Resources_teachers_schools/Drug_Curriculum/Primary/curriculum_gr1to10glossary.html>.

situation in which you have just found yourself. Since raising your blood sugar, heart rate, and alert level likely caused you to use a lot of energy, one of the actions of the cortisol is to increase your hunger. While we may not always realize it because of the initial appetite suppression, after the initial stressor is over we eat more. This can be seen in laboratory experiments in which participants are exposed to stressful situations.[1] It can also be seen in experiments in which participants have their blood cortisol levels and hunger levels measured at the same time.[2] Stress leads to increased hunger, which leads to weight gain. Increased cortisol production is not only associated with weight gain, it is likely the cause of weight gain, as we can see from what happens to people who produce excess cortisol due to an abnormality in the adrenal glands.

Cushing's Syndrome and Severe Obesity

Since the idea that stress leads to weight gain can be controversial, let us look at an example that occurs in nature. Cushing's Syndrome, also called hypercorticism, is a hormonal disorder of very high cortisol levels in the blood. The cause of the

---

[1] Davis, Jeanie. "How You React to Stress May Affect How Your Clothes Fit." WebMD. 4/04/2009 <http://www.webmd.com/news/20010116/how-you-react-to-stress-may-affect-how-your-clothes-fit>.

[2] Gluck, Marci. "Cortisol, Hunger, and Desire to Binge Eat Following a Cold Stress Test in Obese Women With Binge Eating Disorder." Psychosomatic Medicine. 4/04/2009 <http://www.psychosomaticmedicine.org/cgi/content/abstract/66/6/876>.

disorder is an abnormality in the adrenal glands which causes an excess in cortisol production.[1]

The results of the high cortisol levels in Cushing's Syndrome are what we would expect, based on the experiments performed on stress. Symptoms we would predict include increased hunger, rapid weight gain, and obesity. Other symptoms are psychological problems, acne, hypertension, high blood sugar, heart disease, and many more. Fortunately, effective treatments exist to control this disease. When cortisol production returns to normal, hunger and weight levels return to normal as well.

Cortisol and Seasonal Weight Gain

People, especially those at high latitudes, naturally tend to gain fat in the winter and lose it in the summer. While we are often aware of this by looking at our bathroom scales, this seasonal fluctuation can actually be more significant than we realize. We also tend to lose muscle in the winter and gain it in the summer. While we may notice that we have put on five pounds in the winter, we may actually have lost five pounds of muscle and gained ten pounds of fat.

When the body is functioning normally, our blood cortisol levels rise in the winter and fall in the summer, especially in latitudes with more severe winters. This is what is responsible for

---

[1] "Cushing's Syndrome." National Endocrine and Metabolic Diseases Information Service. 4/04/2009 <http://www.endocrine.niddk.nih.gov/pubs/cushings/cushings.htm#causes>.

seasonal weight gain and loss, as well as seasonal mood changes. In people who are overweight, this seasonal cycle is disrupted, with higher levels year round, and especially high levels in the winter. The way the body determines the seasons is not entirely clear. There is some evidence that the clues are visual; in other words, the cycle may depend upon the amount of light that we see throughout the day at different times of the year.

There is also some evidence that vitamin D production plays a role. During the winter a type of ultraviolet light, UVB, is not present at higher latitudes. When this light hits the skin the body is able to manufacture vitamin D from cholesterol, the same substance from which the body manufactures cortisol. During the winter months, when UVB light is not present, vitamin D production drops and this may allow the body to create more cortisol.

This may be part of the reason why Hispanic-Americans have higher cortisol levels than non-Hispanic white Americans and are more likely to be overweight. Increased skin pigmentation blocks UVB rays, lowering vitamin D production, and may allow more cortisol to be produced. On the other hand, decreased vitamin D production may also be a signal to the body that it is winter and it should put on weight. More research is needed before scientists have a definitive answer for what causes these changes. The body likely has more than one influence on its seasonal clock. What we know with certainty is that the seasons, ethnicity, and cortisol all play a role in weight regulation.[1,2]

Stress and Aging

Cortisol's effects on weight are reason enough to want to understand what can make our levels too high, but there is another reason. There is evidence raised cortisol levels increase aging. Every cell contains something called a telomere. A telomere is like a clock; every time a cell divides, a telomere becomes shorter. Shorter telomeres are linked to a range of diseases and aging. A study at the UCLA School of Medicine has shown that higher cortisol levels result in telomeres that become shorter faster. Thus, chronic stress causes our cells to age faster.[3]

Stress in the Modern World

Since we have seen that excessive cortisol levels can cause weight gain by increasing hunger, to stay thin we need to keep our levels normal. This means avoiding stress. It is a cliché that modern life is stressful. Some of the common reasons given for

---

[1] Levine , Matthew. "Diurnal and Seasonal Rhythms of Melatonin, Cortisol and Testosterone In Interior Alaska." Arctic Medical Research. 4/04/2009 <http://www.milliron.net/sad/arcmedres94.htm>.

[2] "Obesity in Minority Populations." American Obesity Association. 4/04/2009 <http://obesity1.tempdomainname.com/subs/fastfacts/Obesity_Minority_Pop.shtml>.

[3] "Study identifies mechanism linking stress to physical illness, aging." UCLA Newsroom. 4/04/2009 <http://newsroom.ucla.edu/portal/ucla/ucla-study-identifies-mechanism-53166.aspx?link_page_rss=53166>.

stress are too many obligations, negative thoughts, working long hours, verbal abuse, and the fast pace of modern life. [1]

We can look at this list and say modern life is indeed very stressful, but why should it be more stressful than life several hundred years ago? In the early Americas, there were no two-day weekends. There was no concept of retirement, because people expected to work until they died. Deaths of both mother and baby were common in childbirth. The number one cause of death was infectious disease, and it was very common for parents to outlive their young children. Yet despite all of this, we still perceive modern life as more stressful than it used to be.

Since many of the things we normally think of as causing stress used to be more common than they are today, it may be that the causes of modern stress and weight gain are physical rather than psychological. Now that we have seen that excess cortisol can cause excess hunger and is the mechanism for weight gain from stress, seasonal changes, and Cushing's Syndrome, it is time to look at what is present in the modern diet that can cause an increase in cortisol levels.

---

[1] Schwartz, Allan. "Anxiety, Worry, and Stress, Oh My: The Bugaboos of Modern Life." Psych Central. 4/04/2009 <http://psychcentral.com/lib/2006/anxiety-worry-and-stress-oh-my-the-bugaboos-of-modern-life/2/>.

Part III: A New Theory of Weight Loss

"The true voyage of discovery consists not of going to new places, but of having a new pair of eyes." -Marcel Proust

Let's review what we know so far. We know that over the last one hundred years changes in our diet—what we call the Western diet—have resulted in more and more Americans becoming overweight. Because of the economic and technological power of the United States, our diet has been spread around the world by international American businesses. This widespread adoption of the Western diet has resulted in increasing levels of obesity in diverse areas of the globe, as a significant percentage of the people who eat this diet gain weight. At the same time, those people who keep their traditional diets remain thin.

While certain people seem to have genes that protect them from becoming overweight on the Western diet, others do not. However, there is still hope for those of us without these genes. We have a mystery, and we need to identify the villain that is causing so much harm to us. Remember our quote from Sherlock Holmes, "Once you eliminate the impossible, whatever remains, no matter how improbable, must be the truth."

If we analyze the components of the Western diet and determine which ones are innocent, whatever remains must contain that which is guilty, no matter how improbable it seems.

If we can identify the culprits that cause weight gain and avoid them, many millions of us can be lean and free of weight gain and the diseases that are associated with it. Here are the main components of the Western diet:

Potential Suspects from the Western Diet

Suspect:	**High Fat Consumption**
Verdict:	Innocent
Reason:	Followers of the Atkins diet showed that, under certain circumstances, high fat consumption doesn't cause weight gain. These people were not genetically prone to being thin, yet they ate a diet consisting largely of meat and fat and became somewhat thinner, at least in the short term. If high fat consumption were the only cause of weight gain, this diet would have made them even more overweight, but it did not. Further evidence against high fat consumption causing weight gain was seen in the French Paradox and Inuit Diet.

Suspect:	**Sugars, Carbohydrates, and Refined Grains**
Verdict:	Innocent
Reason:	If sugary deserts and refined grains were causes of weight gain, the Atkins dieters who avoided them would have become perfectly thin. However, while at one point 10% of North American adults were on the Atkins diet, it later fell from favor, because it did not produce long-term results. Also, we saw that rural Thai have a diet which is calorically 80% white rice, a refined grain, but it is

the urban Thai who have adopted a diet lower in refined carbohydrates who have gained weight.

Suspect: **High Calorie Diet**
Verdict: Innocent
Reason: We saw that normal weight people who volunteered to eat a very high calorie diet, almost 10,000 calories a day in some cases, did gain weight, but when the experiment was over they lost all of the weight without effort. People who had preexisting weight problems but lost weight on a low calorie diet experienced symptoms of starvation when they limited their calories enough to lose weight. Almost all of them regained their weight within three years of losing it.

Suspect: **An Unbalanced Diet**
Verdict: Innocent
Reason: An unbalanced diet may not be healthful, but it is also not the cause of weight gain. In 1900, Americans received the vast majority of their calories from carbohydrates. At that time, only about 1 in 150 people was significantly overweight. It is only as we have started eating more protein and fat that our weight has increased. However, this seems coincidental because protein and fat are also not the cause of weight gain.

With that, it appears that we are at a loss. We know that something in the Western diet is causing weight gain, but all of the traditional suspects are innocent on closer examination.

Scientists as a whole are baffled by this and, without a solution, the problem has become worse and worse. There are now more people in the world who are overweight than who have insufficient food—but there is one thing we are overlooking.

We have ruled out all of the traditional sources of calories in the Western diet, but we have not proved that what causes obesity contains calories. We have made the mistake of assuming this. Remember the research we looked at earlier that we need to explain. We need to explain why soda causes weight gain and why diet soda causes more weight gain than regular soda does. Diet soda has essentially no calories, so whatever is causing weight gain from diet soda doesn't have any calories.

We have to explain the Hunger-Obesity Paradox: Why is it that overweight people have higher levels of hunger than people of normal weight? We have to find out what is causing this greater hunger. We also have to explain why overweight people have higher levels of cortisol secretion and higher cortisol levels in their body tissues, and we have to explain what is causing the higher levels of stress witnessed in people who gain weight.

There is one substance that can explain all these effects. It is something that we have been consuming in gradually increasing amounts for a hundred years, never suspecting that it could cause us to gain weight, and it is now everywhere. We have even tried using it for weight loss.

The Improbable Culprit

The suggestion that caffeine causes weight gain would probably produce in most people an initial reaction that is a cross between condescension and disbelief. That is why the first part of the book was spent learning more about what does not cause weight loss. While we have been taught to think about weight gain as being caused by the types of foods we eat, we have seen example after example that challenges this idea.

We have seen how our hunger level can be changed by medicines that influence hormone production. We have seen the evidence that diets which restrict calories, carbohydrates, and fats do not work. We have seen that exercise is ineffective in causing long-term weight loss. We have seen that our level of cortisol production is key to affecting our hunger level, and that excess hunger can cause weight gain in many instances.

We have seen that increased hunger can explain increased food consumption and weight gain in the United States over the last hundred years, weight gain as a side effect of prescription drugs, weight gain from chronic stress, and weight gain from Cushing's Syndrome. Now we are ready to explore how caffeine could affect our body's hormone regulation in a way that makes excess hunger occur. We will also explore why it is that scientists have overlooked this mechanism for weight gain, and how genetic differences have made it difficult to observe the relationship between increased caffeine consumption and increased obesity.

What Is Caffeine?

We are constantly surrounded by caffeine in our daily lives. In the doses we consume, caffeine is a stimulant that can make us feel more alert and energetic. Most of us simply assume it is as harmless as any other familiar ingredient in our food. It is not; in fact, caffeine is literally a poison. Caffeine is found in the beans, leaves, and fruits of certain plants. It is harmful even to the plants that produce it, which store it in specialized cells that shield the rest of the plant from its harmful effects. Its purpose is to paralyze and kill insects that eat the plant.[1]

Make no mistake; caffeine will kill humans as well.[2] The amount that we consume in our coffee, tea, and soda is highly diluted. However, two grams of pure caffeine over a short period of time, about the weight of five peas, can result in hospitalization, and twenty grams will kill the average adult.

You are unlikely to get a lethal dose from drinking soda, since you would need to drink forty to fifty 32-ounce cups of it all at once. On the other hand, there are certainly many Americans who get that cumulative dose of caffeine in a week, every week. In fact, there have been deaths[3] and hospitalizations of people

---

[1] Rosner, Dalya. "Why Plants Make Caffeine." The Naked Scientists. 4/04/2009 <http://www.thenakedscientists.com/HTML/articles/article/dalyacolumn2.htm/>.

[2] Kerrigan, S; Lindsey T (October 4, 2005). "Fatal caffeine overdose: two case reports" (reprint). Forensic Sci Int. 153 (1): 67–69.

[3] Holmgren, P; Nordén-Pettersson L, Ahlner J (January 6, 2004). "Caffeine fatalities — four case reports" (reprint). Forensic Sci Int. 139 (1): 71–73.

who have taken too many caffeine pills or energy drinks.[1] In its concentrated form, caffeine is quite lethal to humans. Getting a less than lethal dose of caffeine is still associated with a range of negative effects, but right now we will focus on just two that we have already seen can have an effect on weight.

---

[1] Mrvos, RM; Reilly PE, Dean BS, Krenzelok EP (December 1989). "Massive caffeine ingestion resulting in death." Vet-Hum-Toxicol 31 (6): 571–2.

Explaining Current Weight Loss Research

Caffeine has been implicated in a host of disorders, but weight gain is not one of them. This does not mean caffeine is not responsible for weight gain; it just means that we have to look very carefully at the evidence because it is a new theory. First we have to see if caffeine can explain any of the unexplained research on weight gain. Remember, there are four issues that have been associated with weight gain that we haven't been able to fully explain. These are the hunger-obesity paradox, why sleep deprivation predicts weight gain, why regular and diet soda consumption predict weight gain, and the correlation between stress and weight gain. After we examine the role of caffeine in the unresolved issues in weight loss research, we will see whether caffeine consumption can explain modern weight gain.

Caffeine and Stress

Weight gain has been shown to increase in periods of stress. After an initial stressor has passed, our hunger levels are higher than they would otherwise be. Studies have shown that it isn't being overweight that causes stress, but being stressed that leads to becoming overweight.[1] So what is unexplained is why Americans should be more stressed than our ancestors who worried about finding enough to eat.

---

[1] Warner, Jennifer. "Stress Unlocks Fat Cells, Ups Obesity." WebMD. 4/04/2009 <http://www.webmd.com/diet/news/20070702/stress-unlocks-fat-cells-ups-obesity>

Daily caffeine consumption can explain this increased stress. Long-term caffeine use can result in multiple stress hormones becoming elevated, including the hormone cortisol. As explained previously, cortisol is the stress hormone that is also associated with increased hunger. Heightened cortisol production and heightened cortisol tissue levels are found in people who are overweight.[1]

There is the question of how strong the effect of caffeine is on our bodies. Is caffeine's effect strong enough to cause over two-thirds of Americans to be overweight? Is the opposite true, instead, that the amount of caffeine the average American is drinking not strong enough to cause these types of effects? Is there another cause we are missing?

Around 90 percent of Americans consume caffeine every day, whether from soda, coffee, tea, energy drinks, or another source. That makes caffeine America's favorite drug by far. It takes only 200 milligrams (mg) of coffee to measurably increase anxiety levels.[2] More than half of adults in America are consuming more than 300 mg every day. That is enough to cause muscle twitching, irregular heartbeat, nervousness, flushing of the face, what we commonly think of as caffeine jitters, and increased cortisol production. Caffeine is socially acceptable as a drug, so

---

[1] Cherniske, Stephen. *Caffeine Blues*. Grand Central Publishing, 1998. p 61.
[2] "Information about Caffeine Dependence." Johns Hopkins Bayview Medical Center. 4/04/2009 <http://www.caffeinedependence.org/caffeine_dependence.html>.

we have stopped thinking about its consequences.[1] After all, how can caffeine be so bad if we are allowing five-year-olds to drink it in soda? However, this reasoning is faulty. It wasn't too long ago that we placed asbestos in building insulation and lead in paint because we were unaware of the consequences.

There are four caffeine-related psychiatric disorders in the *Diagnostic and Statistical Manual of Mental Disorders*. There have been many cases of anxiety disorders that have been successfully treated simply through caffeine abstention.[2] People who have drunk too much caffeine have been mistakenly admitted to psychiatric hospitals for treatment of anxiety disorders.[3] Clearly, the effect long-term caffeine use has on our bodies can be profound.[4]

Caffeine and the Hunger-Obesity Paradox

Another effect we need to explain is the hunger-obesity paradox. People who are obese tend to experience higher levels of hunger than those who are thin. Since people who are overweight have eaten more than those who are thin have eaten, they should

---

[1] Benjamin, LT Jr; Rogers AM, Rosenbaum A (January 1991). "Coca-Cola, caffeine, and mental deficiency: Harry Hollingworth and the Chattanooga trial of 1911." J Hist Behav Sci 27 (1): 42–55

[2] Snyder SH, Pamela Sklar. Psychiatric Progress: Behavioral and Molecular Actions of Caffeine: Focus on Adenosine. J. Psychiat. Res.1984. 91-106.

[3] Greden JF. Anxiety or Caffeinism: A Diagnostic Dilemma. Amer Journ Psychiatry. 1974. 1089-1092.

[4] Bruce, MS and M Lader. "Caffeine abstention in the management of anxiety disorders." Psychological medicine. Vol. 19, No. 1. Feb. 1989: 211-214.

not be hungrier. This suggests that whatever is causing people to be overweight is causing them to be hungrier.

As we have already discussed, caffeine consumption, especially chronic caffeine consumption, raises levels of the stress hormone cortisol. While we do not always think of stressful situations as causing us to eat more, this is because the initial stressor also releases adrenaline. The adrenaline keeps us from being hungry, but it wears off much faster than the cortisol, so later we eat more. Chronic caffeine use leads to higher production of the hormone cortisol. This causes raised hunger, even when we have eaten enough.

The Hunger-Obesity Paradox is only a paradox when we think of weight gain as having come about because we have chosen to eat too much food. If we think of weight gain as having been caused by caffeine or another substance that disrupts hormone regulation to cause hunger, which then leads to weight gain, hunger and obesity change from paradox to cause and effect.

Caffeine and Sleep Deprivation

Another unexplained predictor of weight gain is sleep deprivation. Chronic sleep deprivation is a feature of modern life and has significant consequences. People who sleep five or fewer hours weigh more than those who sleep seven hours or more.

People who sleep less also tend to gain more weight over time. They are hungrier and crave more sweets.[1,2]

It is possible that sleep deprivation by itself causes these effects, since sleep deprivation causes cortisol levels to spike, but it is also possible that caffeine consumption is causing people to sleep less and have less restful sleep. Caffeine may be a partial explanation for why we are sleeping less in the modern era. Having 200 mg of caffeine in the morning has been shown to measurably interfere with sleep. This is less than the amount of caffeine in a large cup of coffee and is significantly less than the amount of caffeine the average American adult consumes every day.

Just as we usually eat until we are not hungry, we sleep until we are not tired, unless we are awakened prematurely, such as by an alarm clock. While some of us may miss out on sleep during the week, we make up for it on the weekends. Just as eating too much over the long term has a biological cause, sleeping too little over the long term has a biological cause. In laboratory tests people who have been given caffeine before going to sleep exhibit the same symptoms as people suffering from insomnia. With almost 90% of Americans now consuming caffeine daily, it is no wonder that more and more of us are having trouble sleeping.

---

[1] Laino, Charlene. "Sleep Deprivation Linked to Weight Gain." Medscape Medical News. 4/04/2009 <http://www.medscape.com/viewarticle/533105>.

[2] Barclay, Laurie. "Getting Sufficient Sleep May Help Reduce Weight Gain." Medscape Medical News. 4/04/2009 <http://www.medscape.com/viewarticle/495410>.

Since caffeine can cause decreased sleep, the idea that caffeine causes weight gain can explain why people who sleep less gain more weight. Caffeine both interferes with sleep and increases hunger, and increased hunger causes weight gain. This is another example of why correlation does not imply causation. The fact that sleep deprivation and weight gain go together doesn't rule out some third factor, such as caffeine, causing both of them, rather than one causing the other.

However, most of us drink caffeine in the morning to help us function well upon awakening, and there is little evidence that giving up caffeine will enable us to sleep well enough to wake up at sunrise without an alarm clock the way our ancestors did. Caffeine consumption can explain some disruption of sleep, but we are drinking caffeine because we are having difficulty sleeping soundly enough at night to be alert during the day. There is another factor disrupting our sleep cycle, and it is likely that we are drinking caffeine in part to cope with it. We'll examine this other factor in the next chapter.

Caffeine and Soda Consumption

We now return to what was a rather startling study discussed in the previous chapter. Scientists at the University of Texas discovered in an eight-year study that people who drank more soda were much more likely to gain weight than those who drank less. On average, each additional can of diet soda per day increased a person's chance of becoming overweight by about 41%. The reaction to this study was to try to find a reason that artificial sweeteners would cause weight gain. It was not considered surprising that soda made with sugar would cause weight gain, even though we have seen that sugar in juice does not cause weight gain. What we need to do is see if caffeine can explain why both regular soda and diet sodas cause weight gain. As previously presented, here is the data showing the percentages of the normal weight study participants who became overweight or obese, according to their soda consumption.[1]

Consumption	Regular Soda	Diet Soda
up to 1/2 can daily	26.0%	36.5%
1/2 to 1 can daily	30.4%	37.5%
1 to 2 cans daily	32.8%	54.5%
over 2 cans daily	47.2%	57.1%

Looking at the table, we can see that drinking diet soda was about 36% more likely to be associated weight gain than regular soda among the subjects in the experiment. That is an extremely interesting number. The diet version of the best selling soda in the world, whose name will not be mentioned, has 30% more caffeine than its regular version. This degree of difference is only for the most popular soda; the number varies depending on brand and flavor but, if we assume the subjects drank the leading brand of soda, the degree of caffeine difference between regular and diet sodas could explain about 85% of the difference in probability of weight gain between drinkers of the two types of soda studied.

[1] DeNoon, Daniel. "Drink More Diet Soda, Gain More Weight?" WebMD. 4/04/2009 <http://www.webmd.com/diet/news/20050613/drink-more-diet-soda-gain-more-weight>.

There is no other plausible theory that explains why both regular and diet sodas cause weight gain, as well as why diet soda causes even more weight gain than regular soda. Artificial sweeteners or sugar in soda cannot explain the increasing number of overweight people in the modern world, but the idea that caffeine causes weight gain, and soda has been a relatively new way for people to consume caffeine, would explain why the problem of weight gain has become so much worse in recent years. The idea that caffeine causes weight gain would also explain the problem of childhood obesity. While children almost never drink coffee or tea, many children and teenagers are now drinking very large quantities of soda, not to mention caffeine laden "energy drinks."

The Lack of Childhood Obesity in Israel

Incidentally, this theory also explains the relative thinness of Israeli children, giving me one of my final insights into this cause of weight gain. Overall, the percentage of Israelis who are overweight is less than half of that in the United States.[1] While the childhood obesity rate is 16% in the United States, it is almost nonexistent in Israel, particularly in Jerusalem.[2] Young people are thinner even than what is considered normal in the United States. Anecdotally, on a flight out of Tel Aviv, I sat next to a young

---

[1] Sheffer, Rivka . "Trends in overweight, obesity and blood pressure among Israeli working adults—implications for public health." European Journal of Public Health. 4/04/2009 <http://eurpub.oxfordjournals.org/cgi/content/abstract/18/2/121>.
[2] Parker-Pope, Tara. "Hint of Hope as Child Obesity Rate Hits Plateau." New York Times. 4/04/2009 <http://www.nytimes.com/2008/05/28/health/research/28obesity.html>.

Israeli soldier. Her waist was so small that she had trouble adjusting the seat belt so it was tight enough. There was extra room around her hips. She was not particularly thin for an Israeli woman her age, but the seats were not designed for someone with her waist size.

As discussed previously, soda is the number one source of caffeine for children in the United States. American children drink so much soda that it is their primary source of sugar. However, in Israel soda is not available the way it is in the United States. While almost all restaurants in the United States have soda fountains, almost no restaurants in Israel have them. Soda is sold by the can or the bottle, which can cost two or three dollars per serving with no free refills. The few establishments like McDonald's and movie theaters that have soda fountains have much smaller serving sizes. However, this is not the only factor lowering soda consumption among Israeli youth.

My first summer in Israel was spent in Jerusalem, where summers are hot and dry. On many days the temperature reaches over 100 degrees. One of the first things foreign students are told is to always carry a large bottle of water. They are also advised to try to avoid drinking soda because it causes dehydration. In the hot dry summers of Jerusalem, this is a serious threat for young people and tourists who spend most of their time outdoors. Stories of tourists hospitalized because of dehydration are not uncommon.

Because of the high cost of soda, lack of availability, and concern over dehydration among people who spend their days outdoors, soda consumption among Israeli children is much less than among American children. Since children get the vast majority of their caffeine from soda, the children of Israel drink relatively little caffeine. This accounts for the very low rate of childhood obesity. Among Israelis who are older and more likely to have air conditioned cars and office jobs, dehydration is not a concern. Coffee and tea are quite popular among Israeli adults. The theory that caffeine causes weight gain can explain why, while obesity is much rarer among the children of Israel than those in the United States, the gap between adult obesity rates in the two countries is much lower.

Caffeine and Seasonal Weight Gain

Another phenomenon which caffeine may explain is the disruption of the seasonal weight cycle. Humans do not hibernate. We do not retreat into caves and sleep the entire winter, although some of us feel as if we could. However, we are mammals and we have some traits related to those mammals which do hibernate.

In climates far enough away from the equator to have noticeable winters, we experience some of the same things that happen to animals that hibernate. We gain fat and lose muscle in the winter, and we experience greater levels of sleepiness and lethargy. In nature, the weight that we gain in winter should go away in spring, and in summer we should be at our leanest. This is a great defense against starvation in winter, when food is more likely to be scarce, but this mechanism is not serving its natural purpose in the United States. Studies have shown that the majority of our weight gain is still occurring during the winter, but we are not losing it during the rest of the year.[1]

This change in the normal pattern of seasonal weight fluctuation can also be explained by our caffeine-weight gain hypothesis. Cortisol levels are highest in the winter and lowest in the summer. We have seen that cortisol regulates our level of hunger, and cortisol seems to be part of the body's natural way of regulating seasonal changes in our weight. Chronic caffeine use is increasing our cortisol levels year round and can explain why our body's weight regulation mechanism has been disrupted. Our cortisol levels are not falling enough in the summer to lose the body fat we are accumulating in the winter, and we are gaining excess weight.

---

[1] "Holiday Weight Gain Slight, But May Last A Lifetime." National Institutes of Health. 4/04/2009 <http://www.nichd.nih.gov/news/releases/holidayweightgain.cfm>.

The Usual Suspect Revisited

While caffeine's effect on cortisol production offers an explanation for the studies discussed previously, it does not fully explain our sleep disturbances; many people do not consume caffeine yet still do not sleep well enough to wake up easily at an early hour. There is another factor in the modern Western diet which also increases cortisol production and which contributes to this.

The idea that certain types of fats can cause us to gain weight is not controversial in the way the idea that caffeine causes weight gain is. What is not generally recognized is that certain fats can also cause sleep quality to fall and cortisol production to rise in the same manner as caffeine. Giving up caffeine can bring a significant improvement in a person's sleep pattern. However, there is no evidence that this will be sufficient to return one's sleep quality to that of our ancestors; a change in the type of fat consumed may also be needed.

We are all descended from people who woke up early, often at sunrise, feeling refreshed. Indeed, most mammals awaken and sleep with the sun. Today we drink caffeine in order to help us feel alert at an hour when we used to be fully awake. In fact, the biggest problem many people have with quitting caffeine is that they are unable to function in the morning without it. At any coffee house in America, the busiest time of day is the morning rush of people who are on their way to work.

College students, who drink much less coffee than working adults, are also having trouble sleeping. College classes that start before 10:00 a.m. are notoriously under-attended. Students without morning classes are sleeping much later than that hour. When I was an undergraduate at the University of California Santa Barbara, I visited a water treatment plant to study the technology involved in waste water purification. The same plant was also responsible for pumping fresh water into our small college town of Isla Vista. A chart showed that peak water usage, the time when most people woke up and showered, occurred at about noon. Young children, who are the lowest users of caffeine in our society, are also known to have difficulty waking up early. Sleep problems, which are predictors of weight gain, cannot be fully explained by caffeine consumption. While caffeine does appear to contribute to sleep disturbance, fat intake is another factor which we have not yet explored.

The Traditional Explanation of Sleep Disturbance

Of course, it is not a secret that caffeine can disrupt sleep, and people who have difficulty sleeping have already been encouraged to quit caffeine. Many of us continue drinking caffeine because something else in the modern world besides caffeine is impairing our sleep. One common theory is that indoor lighting is responsible. There is some evidence that electric lighting can push back our sleep cycle by about an hour, but there is no evidence that it affects sleep quality. If a lack of intense light in the morning and a lack of darkness at night were responsible for poor sleep quality, then we would expect light therapy to produce improvement. Light therapy involves sitting in front of an intense light box in the morning and avoiding intense light in the evening. The majority of people who try this therapy discontinue it within the first year. The most common treatments for sleep disorders are drugs. This implies that sleep disorders have a biological cause. Since they have become so much more prevalent in recent times, we can assume something in the modern environment is responsible.

Omega-3 Fats

There is a change in the modern Western diet that has been shown to affect sleep quality. From studies of Paleolithic nutrition, hunter-gatherer societies, and pre-industrial societies, scientists know that until the late 19th century omega-3 fats were eaten in equal amounts to omega-6 fats. The current Western diet contains twenty to thirty times the amount of omega-6 fats as omega-3 fats.[1] This high consumption of omega-6 fats, coupled with low consumption of omega-3 fats, has been shown to result in poor sleep quality.[2] Also, omega-3 fats lower cortisol production, just as caffeine raises it. Although omega-3 fats have an effect on sleep opposite from that of caffeine, my personal experimentation shows that the effects of the former do not appear to be sufficient to cancel the sleep disruption caused by the latter.

You may have already heard of omega-3 fats. They have become one of the latest health crazes, and with good reason.

---

[1] Simopoulos, Artemis. "Essential fatty acids in health and chronic disease". American Journal of Clinical Nutrition. 4/24/2009 <http://www.ajcn.org/cgi/reprint/70/3/560S.pdf>.
[2] Yehuda, Shlomo. "Omega-6/Omega-3 Ratio and Brain-Related Functions". Karger Medical and Scientific Publishers. 4/24/2009 <http://content.karger.com/ProdukteDB/produkte.asp?Doi=73791>.

Omega-3 fats have been found to benefit many chronic health conditions that are prevalent in the modern world, including high cholesterol, cardiovascular disease, diabetes, arthritis, psoriasis, acne, and more. It is quite conceivable that the increasing rates of these chronic conditions are, in fact, tied to the lack of omega-3 fats in the modern diet.

Omega-3 from Fish

Wild salmon is one of the most commonly available sources of omega-3 fats in the modern diet. Unfortunately, it can also contain heavy metals and pollutants. However, much of the fish sold in the United States is raised on farms, rather than in the ocean. This farm raised fish is not fed algae, the source from which ocean raised fish acquire omega-3 fats and, as such, contains no omega-3 fats. Farm raised salmon is actually brown instead of pink because of this. It has to be dyed pink to have the look of wild salmon. Restaurants and supermarkets can choose the exact shade of pink that they would like their salmon to be dyed.

Fish oil supplements are a way to avoid farm raised fish, but they can contain the same pollutants and heavy metals as ocean raised fish. They also introduce another danger. Omega-3 fats break down very quickly without refrigeration. One of the reasons the modern Western diet lacks omega-3 fats is that companies which want their products to have a long shelf life avoid using omega-3 fats. Omega-3 pills can start to turn rancid inside the capsule. Eating spoiled fish oil can make you sick rather than healthy.

Despite the difficulty of obtaining omega-3 fats from fish or fish oils, the absence of fish in our diet can't be responsible for deterioration of our health in the modern age, because humans in earlier times did not all eat fish. Before the age of refrigeration, fish was available only to people living near oceans or rivers. In earlier eras, many farming communities were inland, dependent on wells and rain for water, and had no access to fish, yet they had populations that were of similar health to those who lived near the coast. They had another source of omega-3 fat.

Omega-3 from Flax

Flax is the richest plant source of omega-3 fat. If you eat a lot of salad and like the taste of flax seeds or ground flax, including it in your salad can be a good way to get omega-3 fats in your diet. However, flax seed oil is usually recommended as a source of omega-3 fat because it is much more concentrated. While nutritionally it may be healthful, the taste is rather bad. Most people who recommend it suggest drinking it while holding your nose. Also, flax seed oil needs to be refrigerated and often starts to go rancid before being purchased. In addition to this, flax was never a major component of the pre-modern diet, so its absence can't be related to modern health problems.

The Traditional Source of Omega-3 Fats

One of the most profound changes in the modern diet is one that is not obvious from health statistics or the appearance of the food that we eat. While it may not seem significant, the fact that most farm animals are now fed corn and soy, rather than being able to eat grass and hay, has profoundly altered our diet. Before the 20th century, when meat was a luxury consumed mainly by the rich, and the lack of refrigeration and pasteurization made milk consumption much rarer, cheese was much more widely available. Just as fish are a source of omega-3 fats when they eat green algae, cow's milk and cheese are excellent sources of omega-3 fats when the cows are able to eat grass, their natural food source.

No animals are able to independently produce omega-3 fats; we have to get them from a plant source, usually a green plant. Fish get omega-3 fats from algae, cows from grass, and humans from omega-3 rich dairy or fish or from very large quantities of vegetables. Cheese and vegetables were likely our main source of omega-3 fats in pre-modern times. An amount of cheese equivalent in size to a small matchbox provides the recommended daily amount of omega-3 fats, when that cheese is made from the milk of a cow that has been fed only grass.

While many of us may find it difficult or undesirable to eat a largely vegetable based diet, it is rather easy for us to eat small amounts of cheese from pastured cows. Many gourmet cheeses and organic cheeses at health food stores are from cows that are fed solely grass and not commercial feed. Unlike flax seed oil and fish oil capsules, these cheeses are likely to taste very good. Gourmet cheese makers feed their cows grass to improve the taste of their cheese. Another benefit of this source of omega-3 fat is that it is unlikely to be spoiled. Also, while red meat from animals that have been fed grass is high in omega-3 fats, it is significantly more expensive that conventional meat and unlikely to be found in restaurants.

Effects of Omega-3 in Laboratory Experiments

Because most fat in our diet is from animal sources, and the amount of omega-3 fats in animal sources is dependent on what they have been fed, it is very difficult to look at the effects of omega-3 fats on large populations. The records of what animals have been fed over time in different countries are not readily available, so our best source for information about the effects of omega-3 is laboratory experiments. Since we have seen sleeping less causes raised cortisol levels and is a predictor of weight gain, we will focus on the connection between omega-3 fats and sleep. In addition to this connection, there is research concluding that omega-3 deficiency affects a variety of brain functions including memory, learning, mental health, and more.[1]

According to Professor Shlomo Yehuda of Bar Ilan University, "Sleep quality is a major problem in the modern society. Vast numbers of 'healthy people' complain about the quality of their sleep. One of the major complaints is that sleep does not refresh them enough."[2] Professor Yehuda goes on to describe the various studies that show, in both human and rats, improvements in sleep quality, depth of sleep, sleep duration, daytime energy level, and time taken to fall asleep when consumption of omega-3 fats was increased. These improvements occurred in multiple studies. The greatest improvement occurred

---

[1] Yehuda, Shlomo. "Omega-6/Omega-3 Ratio and Brain-Related Functions". Karger Medical and Scientific Publishers. 4/24/2009 <http://content.karger.com/ProdukteDB/produkte.asp?Doi=73791>.
[2] Idem.

in individuals who consumed no more than four times the amount of omega-6 fats as omega-3 fats.[1]

As noted previously, the Western diet contains twenty to thirty times the amount of omega-6 fats as omega-3 fats.[2] Remember, before the late 19th century we consumed these fats in equal amounts. Since consumption of a low ratio of omega-3 to omega-6 fats causes sleep quality to decline, the fat composition of the modern Western diet explains why so many of us can't seem to get up in the morning and feel the need to drink caffeine.

Explaining Our Previous Experiments on Fat

We have seen multiple examples in which high fat consumption has failed to correlate with weight gain. However, our previous analysis of those examples has not taken into account fat type or the effects of caffeine. Recall that the Inuit eating their traditional diet receive 75% of their calories from fat and gain weight only when they eat a lower fat Western diet. However, much of the fat in their traditional diet is of the omega-3 type. Ocean caught fish are high in omega-3 because they feed on algae. Animals, like seals, that feed on these fish are rich in omega-3 fats, as well. While the Inuit consume less fat when they adopt a more Western diet, most of the fat is omega-6 fat, having come from animals that are given feed made from corn and soy.

---

[1] Simopoulos, Artemis . "Essential fatty acids in health and chronic disease". American Journal of Clinical Nutrition. 4/24/2009 <http://www.ajcn.org/cgi/reprint/70/3/560S.pdf>.
[2] Idem.

The French have much higher fat consumption than Americans but much lower rates of obesity. However, the French also eat meat and dairy products with much higher levels of omega-3 fats than those consumed by Americans. French farmers have a long history of associating the quality of meat and dairy with the quality of the ingredients used to produce it. In France, there are 52 different government designations for meat to indicate the type of environment in which it was produced. French farmers believe that quality grassland is needed to produce quality food.[1]

In contrast, the increased fats consumed on the Atkins diet were generally not omega-3 fats. The American diet is proportionally too high in omega-6 fats, and this is the type of fat that Atkins dieters mostly consumed. While the Atkins diet results in higher consumption of this unhealthy ratio of fats, it also involves quitting caffeine.[2] The effect of a high ratio of omega-6 fats to omega-3 fats is to raise cortisol production, which is opposite from the result of giving up caffeine. These opposite effects of the Atkins diet may cancel each other out to some extent. This implies that, in order to lower our cortisol levels enough to lose weight, it may not be sufficient to just quit caffeine. Although people on the Atkins diet did lose weight, they did not become perfectly lean. It seems that the partial success of the Atkins diet

---

[1] "Grass Fed Cattle Can Taste As Good As Grain Fed, Say British Researchers". Scientific Blogging. 4/24/2009 <http://www.scientificblogging.com/news_releases/grass_fed_cattle_can_taste_good_grain_fed_say_british_researchers>.

[2] Urban, Kevin . "The Atkins Diet and Caffeine are Incompatible". Atkins Diet Advisor. 4/24/2009 <http://www.atkins-diet-advisor.com/atkins-diet-and-caffeine.html>.

was due to its insistence on quitting caffeine and not because of its theory that carbohydrates were responsible for weight gain. Its signature endorsement of all types of fats hindered the diet rather than helped it.

While not all fats are unhealthful, the high amount of omega-6 fats in the American diet is. Whenever we look at studies that measure public health in the United States in terms of meat and fat consumption, we are seeing the effects of this high quantity of omega-6 fats. In the United States, those who follow a semi-vegetarian diet have an obesity rate that is about one-quarter less than meat eaters. Those who both follow a vegetarian diet and avoid dairy have an obesity rate that is one-third less than meat eaters.[1] This is not just a correlation relationship. In long-term studies, people who are instructed to eat a low fat diet gain less weight than those who are not.[2] If this high consumption of omega-6 fats and deficiency of omega-3 fats were the only factor in weight gain, low fat diets would have been more successful. The failure to identify caffeine as a factor in weight gain has led to uncertainty as to whether the types of fats in our modern diet are a cause of weight gain.

---

[1] Newby, PK . "Risk of overweight and obesity among semivegetarian, lactovegetarian, and vegan women". American Journal of Clinical Nutrition. 4/25/2009 <http://www.ajcn.org/cgi/content/abstract/81/6/1267>.

[2] Howard, Barbara V. "Low-Fat Dietary Pattern and Weight Change Over 7 Years ". Journal of the American Medical Association. 4/25/2009 <http://jama.ama-assn.org/cgi/content/abstract/295/1/39>.

Explaining the Rise in Obesity over Time

We have seen that the idea that caffeine consumption can cause weight gain can explain some interesting effects in weight loss research, including the hunger-obesity paradox, the correlation between sleep deprivation and obesity, and the association between stress and weight gain. There is one more relationship that caffeine as a source of weight gain can explain, the increasing level of obesity over time. United States obesity levels have been increasing in prevalence, going from a rate of about 0.7% of the population in 1900 to about 34% today. Let's look at how caffeine consumption has changed over the last century and the beginning of the present one.

Soda

In 1900, soda included cocaine and a small amount of caffeine from the coca leaf. Cocaine is a drug that is associated with weight loss rather than weight gain and which has serious health consequences. After 1903, cocaine was removed from soda, but the amount of caffeine was increased. While soda was originally sold in glass bottles, the introduction of soda fountains has led to greater sizes being sold. Soda has transitioned from being a beverage intended for adults to the beverage from which today's American children get the majority of their caffeine.

Innovation has not been limited only to greater sizes. The number of flavors and types of soda available has steadily increased to appeal to greater taste preferences. Diet sodas were made available in 1982 to appeal to the ever-increasing number of Americans trying to lose weight. Diet soda and artificial sweeteners embodied the idea that eating too many calories by choice or mistake caused weight gain. They also conveyed the notion that caffeine, by speeding up our metabolism, would lead to weight loss, as diet sodas can have as much as 30% more caffeine than their regular equivalents.

Coffee

Coffee has been available in the United States since before its founding. The 1773 Boston Tea Party made drinking coffee an act of patriotism, but it was not until the prohibition of alcohol in the 1920s that coffee sales really started to boom in the United States. By 1940, the U.S. was importing about 70% of the world's coffee crop. During World War II, instant coffee was part of the general infantry ration kit, and coffee had to be rationed for the civilian population. Starbucks was founded in 1971 and has driven coffee consumption to steadily increasing heights since then. In 1995, coffee became the world's most popular beverage. Coffee has been made into sweeter forms and attracted younger audiences. It has gone from a beverage consumed in a six-ounce mug to sizes four times as large. It is added to ice cream, candy, and chocolate flavored beverages.[1,2]

During this period of increasing caffeine consumption we have witnessed a continuing increase in the number of overweight

---

[1] "Coffee History." Koffee Korner. 4/04/2009 <http://www.koffeekorner.com/koffeehistory.htm>.
[2] "History of Coffee." Gourmet Coffee Bean Maker. 4/04/2009 <http://www.gourmetcoffeebeanmaker.com/history-of-coffee.php>.

Americans. There have been so many changes in our eating habits and lifestyles in the last century that this one has received scant attention in the search for the cause of our weight gain. However, there is no doubt that steadily increasing caffeine consumption and steadily increasing obesity levels have gone hand in hand.

From all of this discussion, it is apparent that increased caffeine consumption in the modern age offers a plausible theory for all of the unexplained research about weight gain and changes in obesity levels over time. Decreased sleep quality due to deficiency of omega-3 fats can explain why so many of us cannot seem to live without our caffeine. However, while we have seen very strong and compelling evidence that caffeine and omega-3 deficiency cause weight gain, it is still what might be called circumstantial evidence in a court room. Even though we have ruled out other common suspects as sources of weight gain, there may be some other major factor in addition to caffeine and omega-3 deficiency that has not been identified. To prove that these two factors are the primary causes of weight gain in the modern world, we would need to see the majority of overweight people who gave up caffeine and consumed sufficient omega-3 fats become lean.

Losing Weight

Now we have come back to the beginning. We had a question that we needed to answer, "What are the causes of weight gain in the modern world?" We have seen that they have to be components of the Western diet, because immigrants to the United States who maintain their traditional diets do not gain weight the way immigrants who adopt the Western diet do.

We have seen that all the traditional theories of weight gain—too many fats, carbohydrates, sugars, calories, and lack of exercise—do not explain weight gain on closer examination. We have also seen that the effects of caffeine and omega-3 deficiency can explain why people who gain weight have higher levels of hunger, stress, and sleep disturbances. Later, we will also see how genetic differences in our response to caffeine can explain how researchers missed the evidence that caffeine was a cause of weight gain for so long.

In order to subject what we have learned to the ultimate test, we want to use it to lose weight. Actually, what we really want to do is become lean. So it is time to do something that many of us find difficult: It is time to give up caffeine. This includes most soda, coffee, chocolate, and some teas.

Quitting Caffeine

Caffeine is not addictive in the sense that alcohol, cocaine, and various other drugs are addictive. That does not mean it is easy to quit, especially if you have been drinking it for five, ten, twenty years or longer, often every day, often multiple times a day. Ironically, people use caffeine to cope with sleep deprivation that is largely caused by caffeine. Once you have been totally free of caffeine for several months, you will feel much better than when you were drinking caffeine. The hard part is the transition stage.

Quitting Suddenly

There are basically two strategies for quitting caffeine. The first method, used by this author, is quitting all at once. It is not fun for the first few days, and it is probably easiest to begin on a Friday afternoon or Saturday morning. This allows the sleep deficit to be made up over the weekend. Feelings of tiredness are worst in the first few days, but they can last for weeks. Other withdrawal symptoms can include headaches, difficulty concentrating, and muscle pains.

Quitting suddenly means your body has to cope with more intense withdrawal symptoms. While physically this can be more difficult than gradual withdrawal, mentally it can be easier. You make a commitment to yourself that you are through with caffeine and then you stop.

Quitting Gradually

The second method used for quitting caffeine is to gradually reduce consumption. This is the method advocated by Stephen Cherniske in the book *Caffeine Blues*. He advocates quitting caffeine due to its harmful effects, such as mood disturbances, anxiety, disrupted concentration, hypertension, and increased risk of multiple chronic diseases.

If it is difficult to stop consuming caffeine because of the resulting withdrawal symptoms, these can be lessened by making the change gradually. A person drinking four cups of coffee a day can drink three cups of regular coffee a day during the first week, two cups during the second, and one cup in the third. If this pace is too fast, a cup of coffee can be replaced with decaffeinated coffee. Remember that decaffeinated coffee is not caffeine free, and that as we get older our ability to process caffeine decreases. Eliminating caffeine involves giving up both regular and decaffeinated coffee.[1]

Replacing Caffeine

As with quitting any drug, the hardest part of giving up caffeine is staying off it. This is especially true of caffeine because it is everywhere, even more so than alcohol. It is socially acceptable to drink it at every meal out, every morning at work. In fact, there is almost no time it is not acceptable to use caffeine. Certain coffee chains even have more than one store in the same building. Soda machines are inside schools and hospitals. It is often easier to find a coffee machine than a drinking fountain.

Not being able to order a tasty drink at a meal out with friends while they are all drinking soda, coffee, and tea may feel

[1]Cherniske, Stephen . *Caffeine Blues: Wake Up to the Hidden Dangers of America's #1 Drug.* Grand Central Publishing, 1998.

like a punishment. Often it seems strange. We are expected to drink something when we go out. While water is always available, some people feel as if they are being "cheap" if they order water when they go to a restaurant. Remember, just because you are trying to lose weight does not mean you can't drink something sweet. Most restaurants sell 100% fruit juice without caffeine, although it is necessary to be careful because they may be offering caffeinated fruit punches instead. Juice has become much less popular because of the belief that sugar causes weight gain but, according to the research we saw earlier, 100% fruit juice and sugar are not the cause of weight gain. There are herbal teas that are naturally caffeine free, as opposed to decaffeinated teas which still have some caffeine. Also, while they are not particularly nutritious or healthful, there are caffeine free sodas. Actually, after giving up caffeine for long enough, many people find they lose their taste for soda. The appeal of the soda was caffeine all along.

Measuring Fat Loss

Becoming lean is synonymous with "losing weight," but what we really want to do is lose fat. Caffeine is a diuretic; it causes our bodies to hold less water than normal. As a result, when we quit, we can gain water weight but become leaner. Also, as men lose fat, their estrogen levels decline, and this can cause an increase in lean body mass. Therefore, to measure our initial progress in becoming lean, we need to measure our fat levels, not our overall weight. The easiest way to do this is by measuring our waist.

Most of this book has used the body mass index (BMI) to

describe body fat levels. This is an imperfect measure, especially for men. Women experience much wider changes in BMI than men, because men have a much larger ability to adjust their lean muscle mass in relation to their body fat levels. While the ratio of our waist to our height is a much better measure of body fat, it isn't widely used in research studies. To track individual progress, measuring waist circumference will provide the best measure of fat loss. A decrease of one inch in waist circumference corresponds with a loss of six to eight pounds of fat.

You don't need a scale and you don't need a tape measure. What you need is a belt, one that fits snuggly. Try it on now and take note of the notch where it fits. As you lose weight you will be able to close the belt more. If you lose seven pounds of fat and gain seven pounds of muscle, your scale will tell you that you are not losing weight. However, since muscle is much denser than fat and is not concentrated at the waist, your belt will close another notch. In a few months, you may even fit into smaller pants.

This example is more appropriate for a man than a woman, for as women become leaner their weight falls proportionately more than it does in men. Despite this, women can still measure their fat loss more accurately by looking at their waist circumference rather than at their weight, especially considering the water weight that can be gained when initially quitting caffeine.

The Speed of Fat Loss

We have different susceptibility to the effects of caffeine for genetic reasons, so it is likely we will recover from it at different rates. In *Caffeine Blues*, Stephen Cherniske notes that people recovering from caffeine can notice decreasing stress and anxiety levels over a period of many months. Since stress is associated with increased hunger, it can take months for hunger levels to completely return to normal as well. Assuming there is nothing else in addition to caffeine raising your hunger and stress levels, such as certain prescription drugs, there should be a significant improvement after the first month. To measure your progress, track your waist measurements monthly. Take notice of how your clothes fit, how relaxed you are. In addition to looser clothes, you may realize that your energy level and mood are improving.

Not Needing Caffeine

Of course, we also need to address the underlying reason why many of us feel the need to consume caffeine. We are no longer waking up early in the morning, without an alarm clock, feeling refreshed and ready to go about our day. Since this is likely a result of an unhealthy ratio of omega-3 to omega-6 fat consumption, we can improve our sleep quality by increasing our intake of omega-3 fats and decreasing our intake of omega-6 fats. This means daily consumption of cheese, dairy, or meat from grass fed animals. It also likely means a reduction in consumption of conventional red meats, fried foods, corn oil, and soy oil. At restaurants, omega-3 rich food sources are rarely available, but we can eat more healthful alternatives—foods cooked in canola or olive oil, lean meats, fruits, and vegetables—advice that probably sounds familiar as conventional wisdom on health. Experiment with the omega-6/omega-3 fat ratio in your diet to see what gives you the ideal quality of sleep and reduces your need for caffeine.

Being Overweight Means Being Unhealthy

Worldwide, it is estimated that over one billion people are now overweight.[1] These are shocking numbers, and all the more so when you consider that four or five generations ago there wasn't even an idea that obesity could ever become a major health problem except for a few rare cases. Being overweight was something that afflicted only the very rich, and two hundred years ago it was so rare as to be considered a status symbol. Today, close to one-sixth of the world's population is overweight, a number greater than those who are in danger of not having enough food.[2]

The Harmful Effects of Being Overweight

It was not too long ago that fat cells were looked upon as inactive, their only function being to store energy for a later time when it might be needed. We now know that this was incorrect. In fact, fat cells are closely tied in with our immune system. Rather than simply being passive stores of calories, they also provide powerful feedback to the body regarding how much energy they are storing.

---

[1] "Worldwide overweight and obesity problem 'staggering'." United Nations News Center. 4/04/2009 <http://www.un.org/apps/news/story.asp?NewsID=15937&Cr=health&Cr1=>.

[2] Rosen, Stacey . "Obesity in the Midst of Unyielding Food Insecurity in Developing Countries." Amber Waves. 4/04/2009 <http://www.ers.usda.gov/AmberWaves/September08/Features/ObesityCountries.htm>

Our bodies are used to being in two states, normal weight or underweight. For most of human history, this was all our bodies had to contend with. In the first state, our fat cells would be in what we would think of as a Goldilocks state, not too large and not too small. In the underweight state, our fat cells would be too small. In this case, the body's greatest concern was that it was in danger of starving. To extend its life as long as possible, ideally until more food was available, the body would decrease the activity of the immune system. This would save substantial energy and might prevent death from starvation. It is also why disease follows soon after the onset of famine. Most of the illnesses that ensue are what are known as opportunistic infections, things that can harm the body only when the immune system is in a weakened state.

When starvation is at the door, a weakened immune system is the best of bad options for the body. When enough food becomes available, our fat cells go back to normal size. As they do, our immune system returns to normal levels of functioning. On the other hand, what if we don't just return to normal weight levels? What if we keep eating and we become overweight? Unfortunately, this is a very recent situation for our bodies, and our genes have not had time to adapt to this new situation. Perhaps for this reason, and as a consequence of the mechanism that defends against starvation, as our fat cells enlarge past normal size, our fat cells send signals to the body to keep increasing the level of immune system activity, and we get excess inflammation.

The Link Between Obesity and Chronic Disease

It has long been known that being overweight increases a person's risk for chronic disease, and we know now that inflammation plays a large role in this. The fat that surrounds the organs in the gut, called visceral fat, secretes an inflammatory molecule known as interleukin-6 (IL-6) into the blood. Increases in IL-6 are also associated with another inflammatory substance called C-reactive protein (CRP). High levels of these inflammatory substances over a long period of time are associated with heart disease, cancer, insulin resistance, hypertension, arthritis, type 2 diabetes, and more. As we have become overweight starting in the 20th century, we have experienced much higher rates of these chronic diseases.[1]

Costs to Society

An overweight population causes huge costs to society, due to the higher prevalence of these chronic diseases. It is something we feel in our pocketbook through lower wages for all workers. It has been claimed that pay for middle class workers (adjusted for inflation) has not been increasing over the last forty years, but this is not entirely true. Cash wages haven't been increasing, but overall compensation, including employer costs for health care, has skyrocketed. This can be traced not to prescription drugs, but to the increased use of medical services. Some of this is due to the

[1] Dryden, Jim. "Belly fat may be linked to systemic inflammation." Record. 4/04/2009 <http://record.wustl.edu/news/page/normal/8990.html>.

development of new medical procedures, but there is no doubt that more of these procedures are being performed because of the higher rates of chronic disease. Such diseases become much more prevalent in an overweight population than in one of normal weight.

Not everyone is in favor of government-paid health care, but certainly we would all very much like it if we could make quality health care affordable to more people. Making our entire population free from obesity would drastically drop the costs of providing comprehensive medical insurance. The health care system would become much less burdened because of lower rates of chronic disease.

Not only would a healthier population lead to a huge decrease in our health care costs, it would give doctors the time to practice a better kind of medicine. Physicians are some of the most highly trained and educated people in our society. Imagine the increase in the quality of care if they were not trying to see a new patient every fifteen minutes. Doctors could devote more attention to maximizing patient wellness instead of having barely enough time to deal with the most pressing symptoms of disease.

The Effects of Genetic Diversity

The genes that protect against obesity have not all been identified, much less understood, so we really can't say how they work. There are some things we do know with certainty from observation. We know that excess cortisol can lead to obesity because people with Cushing's Syndrome, who develop adrenal tumors which cause excess cortisol to be produced, experience high levels of hunger and develop obesity. When those tumors are removed and cortisol production returns to normal, the excess hunger and obesity go away. We also know that in many people extended caffeine use leads to stress, sleep deprivation and, eventually, increased cortisol production. However, these effects of caffeine do not occur in a significant minority of the American population. There is a genetic basis for caffeine tolerance and these genes appear to be related to those involved in governing the circadian rhythm.

The Circadian Rhythm

The circadian rhythm is a 24-hour cycle or clock possessed by plants, animals, and certain microbial life. It is made of two processes that oppose each other, one that tells us to be increasingly awake, and the other that tells us to be increasingly asleep.[1] The cycle corresponds with biochemical and behavioral

---

[1] Cromie, William. "Human Biological Clock Set Back an Hour." Harvard University Gazette. 4/04/2009 <http://www.hno.harvard.edu/gazette/1999/07.15/bioclock24.html>.

changes within living beings. In humans, the circadian rhythm governs our sleep-wake cycle, cell regeneration, hormonal changes throughout the day, and our levels of hunger. It is thought that this cycle has been with us from the emergence of the earliest cells. During the day, particularly around noon, high levels of ultraviolet radiation from the sun penetrate the atmosphere. This radiation can severely damage the DNA of single celled organisms, so their DNA replication occurs at night.

There are two ways that our body receives information about the presence of the sun. The first is through our eyes; we see light outside and this tells our body that it is daytime. In fact, according to some researchers, using electric lighting in the evening interferes with the circadian rhythm, causing us to go to sleep later. For the most part, though, the low intensity of indoor lighting is not great enough to have a major effect on our circadian rhythm. Sunlight also influences our body's clock through our skin, where it plays a role in the production of vitamin D.

Adenosine

Adenosine is a biological chemical used by the body in the sleep-wake cycle. When the body is overworked, it releases adenosine to trigger sleep. Adenosine levels spike during sleep deprivation and fall as we sleep. It has been theorized that this is the body's way of tracking the "sleep deficit." Adenosine is also involved in the body's seasonal response. Adenosine levels are higher than normal during the winter in most people. This is related to why we tend to have less energy in the winter than in the summer.

How Caffeine Works

It is not known with absolute certainty how caffeine works. However, the popular theory is that it is through caffeine's effect on the A2a adenosine receptors, one of the four known groups of sensors in the brain for detecting adenosine.[1] To these adenosine receptors, caffeine may look like adenosine because both caffeine and adenosine belong to the same chemical family. It is hypothesized that caffeine works by attaching to the A2a adenosine receptors and blocking adenosine from signaling to the body to become tired.[2]

Scientists have several pieces of data that support this hypothesis. One is that in humans who have a gene associated with an altered A2a adenosine receptor, both anxiety and sleep deprivation from caffeine consumption are inhibited.[3,4] Another piece of data is that mice which have been engineered to have an inhibited A2a receptor appear not to be affected by caffeine.[5] These data are not conclusive because we don't know if altering

---

[1] "Overworked brains release adenosine to slow cells, trigger sleep." Medical News TODAY. 4/04/2009 <http://www.medicalnewstoday.com/articles/23184.php>.
[2] Bryant, Charles. "How Caffeine Works." How Stuff Works. 4/04/2009 <http://health.howstuffworks.com/caffeine3.htm>.
[3] Retey, J V. "A Genetic Variation in the Adenosine A2A Receptor Gene (ADORA2A) Contributes to Individual Sensitivity to Caffeine Effects on Sleep." Clinical Pharmacology & Therapeutics. 4/04/2009 <http://www.nature.com/clpt/journal/v81/n5/abs/6100102a.html>.
[4] "The genetic basis for caffeine-induced anxiety discovered". Science Blog. 4/04/2009 <http://www.scienceblog.com/community/older/2002/F/2002210.html>.
[5] Mobbs, Charles. "Caffeine and the adenosine receptor: Genetics trumps pharmacology in understanding pharmacology." Cellscience. 4/04/2009 <http://www.cellscience.com/Reviews5/caffeine_adenosine_receptor.html>.

genes associated with the A2a adenosine receptor has caused other changes we aren't aware of in both mice and in humans. Even though we are not absolutely certain about the mechanism by which caffeine works, we do know the genes that we associate with the A2a adenosine receptor constitute a biological basis for caffeine tolerance.

Caffeine Tolerance

Genes that prevent caffeine from causing increased stress and sleep deprivation are very valuable to us now. Both increased stress and sleep deprivation lead to weight gain because of their effect on cortisol production. However, caffeine has become widely used only in the last hundred years, and we have no records or even legends that suggest that there was ever a time before the last hundred years that weight gain was a problem for a significant number of people. Throughout our history we have been very lean, and the danger has been starvation rather than excess weight.

In order for a gene to become widespread, it has to convey some type of benefit that makes survival more likely. Therefore, we would not expect a large percentage of people to have genes that protect them against gaining weight when exposed to caffeine. This means these genes must exist because they provide some other benefit. If we can figure out who is more likely to have these genes, we may be able to guess at their original function.

Fortunately, we can identify the people who have a high tolerance to caffeine consumption: They are the very same people who drink large amounts of caffeine. One study of fraternal and identical twins found that genes could predict up to 77% of the likelihood that an individual would be a heavy caffeine user.[1] After all, if caffeine causes you to have difficulty sleeping and to feel anxiety, you are unlikely to be able to drink a very large amount. If drinking large amounts of caffeine makes you feel good, you are likely to drink more.

The World's Heaviest Caffeine Users

The average American drinks the caffeine equivalent of about two cups of coffee a day. That is an amount that can interfere with sleep, and individuals who are sensitive to caffeine have to limit their consumption so as not to have difficulty sleeping. While the people of the United States consumed an average of 4.2 kilograms (kg) of coffee each (or per capita) in 2003, the people of Finland consumed 11.4 kg.[2] The latter amount is equivalent to about five cups of coffee per person per day, and it is only one component of caffeine in the Finnish diet, which includes soda and tea. The people of the Northern European countries are the heaviest coffee consumers in the world. In 2003 the per capita coffee consumption of Iceland was 9.1 kg, of Norway 9.0 kg, of Denmark 8.1 kg, and of Sweden 7.9 kg. Additional caffeine was also consumed in soda and tea.

---

[1] Kendler, Kenneth. "Caffeine Intake, Tolerance, and Withdrawal in Women: A Population-Based Twin Study." American Journal of Psychiatry. 4/04/2009 <http://ajp.psychiatryonline.org/cgi/content/full/156/2/223>.

[2] "Earth Trends Environmental Information." World Resources Institute. 4/04/2009 <http://earthtrends.wri.org/>.

When soda consumption is taken into account, every person in Finland is drinking the equivalent of over six cups of coffee a day. These per capita calculations include children and babies who aren't drinking coffee, so adult coffee consumption is in fact above six cups of coffee per day. We have seen that individuals who drink large amount of coffee are on average those who have higher tolerance to it. This same principle should apply at the national level. The people of the Northern European countries are able to consume this high level of caffeine because they enjoy it. It causes them to feel elated and energetic rather than sleep deprived and stressed. As people in Finland are fond of saying, "We love our coffee." While it is not certain, if the genes which produce caffeine tolerance are concentrated in Northern Europe, it tends to suggest that they are an adaptation to living at high latitude. This is an area for future research to investigate.

Genetic Resistance to Winter Depression

Known adaptations to high latitude in Northern Europeans include light skin and blue eyes. However, there is also an adaptation that prevents winter depression, a condition that is associated with stress, anxiety, and increased cortisol production, which are some of the same symptoms experienced after caffeine consumption. Winter depression, or in medical terms seasonal affective disorder (SAD), has a biological basis. Negative symptoms of SAD also include weight gain, depression, sleep disturbance, and drowsiness. Sufferers are also more likely to report increased levels of hunger and cravings for sweets.

People from northern latitudes have developed genes that protect them against this condition. Among the Caucasian population of Canada, immigrants of Icelandic ancestry have almost 90% lower levels of SAD than the general population. The populations of the Scandinavian countries also have extremely low rates of SAD for their latitude.[1] Since SAD is associated with anxiety, stress, and high cortisol production, the genes that prevent these symptoms from occurring in excess as a response to caffeine may have come about because of their ability to keep these very symptoms from occurring in excess during the winter. It is another area for future research.

Tying it All Together

If the genes that prevent obesity are an adaptation to seasonal affective disorder at high latitudes, it could provide an explanation for the different rates of obesity among ethnic groups. Much more research on the genes that protect against weight gain and seasonal affective disorder needs to be done. Still, knowing that many of us have genes that can protect against obesity in this manner answers an important question: Why has medicine provided us with few solutions for the increasing levels of weight gain over the last one hundred years? The uneven distribution of the genes that protect against weight gain has interfered with scientists' ability to make comparisons between and among different populations, since what makes one group of people gain weight may have no effect on another.

---

[1] Whitehead, Barry S. "Winter Seasonal Affective Disorder: A Global, Biocultural perspective." University of Alabama. 4/04/2009 <www.as.ua.edu/ant/bindon/ant570/Papers/Whitehead.pdf>.

Genetic Differences and Obesity Studies

Obesity is a medical problem that has resulted in so much damage, disease, and death that the idea that scientists have just missed the fact that caffeine contributes to obesity seems unlikely. This should give us some pause. If all we have to do to lose weight is to stop drinking caffeine, then why has no one figured this out?

The information about how much caffeine the people in each country consume has been available for years. Furthermore, if we want to compare the differences among individuals in the same country, we can simply ask them. Most people are quite willing to help medical researchers in this way. If all of us reacted to caffeine in the same way, this problem would have been easy to solve. However, since our response to caffeine depends upon our genetics, solving the obesity puzzle gets more complicated.

Genetic Complications in Studies of Individuals

There has been previous research that has studied potential links between coffee and obesity, between soda and obesity, and between caffeine and obesity. Results have been contradictory, but this tells us more about the way the studies have been conducted than it does about caffeine itself. Scientific studies can be tripped up in a lot of ways. The fact that many of us have a gene that alters the effect caffeine has on us interferes with the data we get from trying to study the effects of caffeine consumption. Most of the research on obesity has been conducted on ethnic Europeans, who appear to be more likely to have the genes responsible for caffeine tolerance. Remember, in all of these studies of caffeine, scientists have not screened out those people who have the gene that inhibits caffeine's ability to affect our stress response. The University of Texas study on soda consumption may have done this sort of genetic screening to some extent, although unintentionally, by including a large number of Mexican Americans.

If you like coffee, soda, or tea, and you have a gene that allows you to drink significant amounts without feeling negative effects, you are likely to drink more than a person who does not have that gene. Consequently, in a study of coffee consumption, more people who have that gene are going to be in the group that drinks large amount of coffee than in the group that drinks medium or small amounts of coffee. The result is that in many of these studies the people who drink moderate amounts of coffee weigh more than the ones who drink lots of coffee or no coffee. Researchers have seen this as evidence that caffeine promotes weight loss, which is why diet drinks and diet pills have caffeine in them. It is only recently that we have discovered the genetic differences in the way people process caffeine, and these genetic differences have not been taken into consideration in any of the studies of the effect of caffeine on weight.

Studying Differences Between Countries

Just as genetics can affect a study of individuals, it can affect a study of countries. Remember how scientists originally tried to prove that fat was the cause of obesity. They looked at the fat consumption of different countries, and they looked at the percentage of people who were overweight. What they saw was that, as fat consumption increased, most of the time the number of people who were overweight increased.

There were some exceptions to this pattern, such as the French and the people of the Northern European countries, who were not as fat as would have been predicted in this model. While this relationship between fat consumption and weight gain seemed to hold true for the most part, these exceptions cast doubt on the belief that one must cause the other. In fact, when we examined people who followed low fat or high fat diets, we found that fat did not cause weight loss or weight gain at all. This situation brings us to the discussion of a well-known mistake in science.

The Classic Mistake of Correlation and Cause

The saying "correlation is not cause" is famous in the mathematical field of statistics. This is the field that is responsible for interpreting and understanding massive amounts of numerical data that can be used in research. What the phrase means is that the fact that two things initially appear to be related does not mean that one causes the other.

The classic example is from a study of storks and newborn babies. Storks are the birds from the children's fable, the birds that are supposed to deliver newborn babies to their parents. It was once discovered by scientists in a certain town that homes with a newborn baby were much more likely to have a nest of storks on their roof. In fact, the number of storks on the roof seemed to be the highest when closest to the day on which a new baby had been delivered.

Obviously, this did not mean that storks were really delivering newborn babies to their parents, as the researchers were no doubt aware. What was actually happening was that houses with newborn babies were much more likely to have lit fireplaces. The storks were nesting on the roofs of houses with newborn babies, not because they had delivered the babies, but because these were the houses with more lit fires, and the storks liked the warmth from the fireplaces that came up through the chimneys. Because we knew how babies were really made, we knew that the storks nesting in the roof were not responsible for their delivery.

On the other hand, since we did not know how people became fat, we did wrongly interpret the relationship between two separate variables. We saw that a country consuming more fat was more likely to have an overweight population. We assumed this meant the people were more overweight because they consumed that fat. However, having a higher wealth level enables consumption of greater amounts of both fat and caffeine. The wrong conclusion was drawn from the data.

The International Genetic Complication

There is no common example for the opposite of the famous statement, which is that lack of correlation is not lack of cause. When we study the differences among countries, we assume that if two countries follow exactly the same diet they should get the same result, but this is not the case. Countries can contain diverse ethnicities and genetic variations of which we are not even aware.

While the genetic differences among all humans are extremely minor, they are enough to make it so that disease prevalence is dissimilar in various ethnic groups. Research from the U.S. National Institutes of Health shows that non-Hispanic white women are more likely to develop osteoporosis than African-American women, and African-American women are more likely to become overweight than non-Hispanic white women. Indeed, there are genetic differences that create different probabilities that people descended from Europe, Latin America, Africa, South Asia, and Japan will become overweight.[1,2]

To see how these differences have hurt researchers' efforts to find the cause of obesity, let us assume we are studying whether caffeine is the main cause of obesity in the modern world and that the genes that prevent weight gain also increase tolerance to caffeine, but we do not know this. We are investigating two types of developed countries, one whose population is genetically unable to gain weight and one whose is, but we do not know this either. People in the first type of country, who are unable to gain weight, are consuming about twice as much caffeine as are people in the second type of country, who are becoming fat. We would

---

[1] "Ancestry and Obesity." Science Central. 4/04/2009 <http://www.sciencentral.com/articles/view.php3?language=english&type=article&article_id=218392039>.

[2] Sample, Ian. "Gene sequence puts half of UK population at greater risk of obesity, researchers say." Guardian. 4/04/2009 <http://www.guardian.co.uk/science/2008/may/05/genetics.health>.

look at the prevalence of obesity and the amount of caffeine consumed. We would see that the populations which are consuming more caffeine are thinner, and we would incorrectly assume that consuming more caffeine is causing them to be thinner. While this scenario may be hypothetical, it is an example of how scientists studying the differences among populations are often unaware of their genetic differences or the effects of those differences.

Genetics have, in fact, interfered with scientists' ability to pinpoint the cause of obesity. The United States has the highest rate of obesity of any country in the world. We know that genes are not responsible for our obesity, because about one hundred years ago almost all Americans were lean. So we are doing something that is causing us to gain weight. However, the Swedes and Norwegians drink more coffee than we do, the French eat more meat and fat, and the Thai eat more refined carbohydrates, all without having the sort of national obesity problem found in the United States today. Because we cannot adjust for differences in genes, we have been unable to use statistics to determine the cause of obesity the way we have used them to solve so many seemingly more difficult problems. By contrast, when we study a chemical substance, like water, every molecule is the same. The first molecule reacts the same way the second does.

In our discussion of the various factors that could be causing us to gain weight, we have ruled out most of the suspects. The only remaining possibility is caffeine, which can lead to weight gain by increasing our level of hunger. This doesn't prove that caffeine is the main source of weight gain in the modern world.

There are prescription drugs that can cause weight gain by increasing hunger and there may be other unknown factors that do this as well. However, all the evidence points to something in our diet being responsible for obesity. Because of the failure to consider the effects of genetic differences in studies that compare rates of caffeine consumption and obesity, caffeine has remained the one component of the Western diet that has never been widely suspected of being a cause of obesity, even after researchers have ruled out all of the other components of that diet. The theory that caffeine causes obesity may seem improbable, but it is one of the few theories that have not been disproved by large numbers of individuals testing it. Future research on the effect of caffeine on obesity will have to take into account the genetic factors that protect many of us from its negative effects.

Final Thoughts

All truth passes through three stages. First, it is ridiculed. Second, it is violently opposed. Third, it is accepted as being self-evident. –Arthur Schopenhauer

If we accept the quote from Arthur Schopenhauer about the three stages of truth, then we are a long distance away from the time when the theory that caffeine can be a cause of obesity is accepted as being self-evident. So how can we move forward from the stage at which the ideas that caffeine can cause weight gain, and omega-3 deficiency fuels caffeine consumption, are ridiculed to the stage at which they are accepted as being self-evident? Socrates, who was known as the wisest man in ancient Athens, may be able to help us. Socrates said, "Let him that would move the world, first move himself." In other words, many people are not likely to be convinced by any argument on this subject. If this includes you, I would point out that you have nothing to lose by giving quitting caffeine a try and much to gain. Eating more omega-3 and fewer omega-6 fats will make this easier. You will save money and sleep better by giving up coffee and soda, and you will have the potential to improve your own health and, eventually, the health of those around you.

Best of luck in both,

Daniel Matthew Korn

Printed in the United States
144441LV00001B/79/P

9 780615 290089